THE
NEW
DIABETIC
C·O·O·K·B·O·O·K

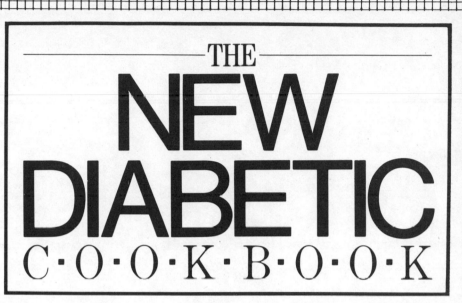

THE
NEW
DIABETIC
C·O·O·K·B·O·O·K

MABEL CAVAIANI

CB

CONTEMPORARY
BOOKS
CHICAGO

Published by Contemporary Books, Inc.
Two Prudential Plaza, Chicago, Illinois 60601-6790
Manufactured in the United States of America
International Standard Book Number: 0-8092-4251-6

For my godchild, Vicki Riley Glastetter,
who has always been a joy to me

CONTENTS

FOREWORD BY DR. CROCKETT

There are estimated to be approximately 11 million persons in America with diabetes—and about 5 million of these people are unaware of having the disease.

The most usual form of diabetes is diabetes mellitus, which has both metabolic and vascular components that are interrelated. The metabolic component is related to a deficiency of insulin activity and is associated with hyperglycemia and altered fat and protein metabolism. Vascular components consist of a speed-up of fatty deposits in the blood vessels and changes in the kidney and eye blood vessels. Treatment of diabetics aims to keep the blood sugar as close to normal as possible. This requires maintaining a balance between diet, insulin, and exercise.

Most people are aware of the importance of diet in the treatment of diabetes. In fact it is possible to completely control the milder forms of diabetes with diet alone without added insulin. The usual diet for diabetics is a balance of carbohydrates, fats, and proteins specifically computed for each individual. It is extremely important that an individual adhere closely to the given diet in addition to eating at regular intervals. It is also important that the individual exercise and maintain a normal weight for his or her sex, type, and build.

There has been much research done in the last few years on the components of diabetic diets. These researchers recommend that the old diabetic diets be changed to include more carbohydrates of the polysaccharides type and less fat of the saturated type. The revised guidelines of the American Diabetes Association recommend that 12 to 20 percent of total calorie intake be protein, 50 to 60 percent be carbohydrate, and up to 20 percent be fat (restricting saturated fats to no more than half). They also suggest restricting cholesterol and saturated fats and substituting unsaturated fats to slow down the progression of atherosclerosis. These guidelines allow more carbohydrate and less fat than previous diabetic diets. Monosaccharides and disaccharides (glucose and sucrose) should be avoided because they are absorbed rapidly after meals and cause increased blood sugar levels; complex carbohydrates, such as starches, are preferred. The American Diabetes Association also suggests that high-fiber, unrefined carbohydrates be substituted for highly refined carbohydrates with low fiber content. The addition of dietary fiber reduces blood sugar levels after meals. The British Diabetes Association basically agrees and also discourages high salt intake to help control cardiovascular complications.

Recommendations on diet alone will be useless if the person does not comply. The diets must be acceptable to individuals in terms of both palatability and the availability of the foods. Diets should interfere as little as possible with the dietary habits of the individual.

This new book by Mabel Cavaiani is a compilation of recipes for use by diabetics. She has taken many commonly known recipes and adapted them to comply with the latest recommendations of the American Diabetes Association and the American Dietetic Association. Her recipes replace much of the monosaccharides and disaccharides with polysaccharides, increase the amount of dietary fiber, decrease the amount of salt, and replace the cholesterol and saturated fats with unsaturated fats. In the process she has brought much more interesting variety into the restrictive diet of diabetics.

—Joseph Turner Crockett, M.D., L.F.A.P.A.
San Diego, California

ACKNOWLEDGMENTS

I would like to thank the following persons for their encouragement and professional help in developing and writing this book. Without their support I could never have written it.

Dr. Susan Urbatsch, of the Medical Clinic, West Union, Iowa, my family doctor. Her wise counsel, care, and concern have helped me learn about and cope with my diabetes.

Mr. Frank Gayda, Chief of the Dietary Department, Holy Cross Hospital, Chicago, Illinois; Mary Agnes Jones, Chief Administrative Dietitian; and the other dietitians on the staff. Their frank appraisal of the need for this book encouraged me to write it; their support helped me to complete it.

Muriel Urbashich, R.D., Director of the Dietary Department of South Chicago Community Hospital, Chicago, Illinois, and her staff. Their generous cooperation and their faith in this cookbook have been an inspiration to me.

Nancy Johnson, R.D., Assistant Director of the Dietary Department, South Chicago Community Hospital, for her frequent help with the therapeutic problems I encountered while writing this book.

Dorothy Berzy, R.D., clinical dietitian at South Chicago Community

Hospital, for her particular help with the chapter on calculating food exchanges.

Mabel Frances Gunsallus, R.D., M.S., Miami, Florida, who spent many hours discussing the theory, recipes, and contents of this book with me. Her continued belief in my professional competence has meant a great deal to me.

Edith Robinson, R.D., M.S., Decatur, Georgia, who shared her knowledge of the low cholesterol diet and encouraged me to put it all down on paper.

Eva Burrack, Food Service Supervisor at the Lutheran Nursing Home and Gernand Retirement Center, Strawberry Point, Iowa, and her dietary staff, for their frank and constructive comments on the many recipes in this book which we taste-tested together.

Mary Klicka, R.D., M.S., Chief of the Ration Design and Evaluation Branch, Food Technology Division, Food Engineering Laboratory, U.S. Army Natick Research and Development Center, Natick, Massachusetts, who helped me with the nutritive information I needed to calculate recipes in this book.

Frances Lee, R.D., M.S., Dietary Consultant of Kerens, Texas (formerly Chief of the Experimental Kitchens, U.S. Army, Natick, Massachusetts), who was always so generous with her help whenever I called with a problem in developing a recipe.

"Chef Dave" Hutchins, Owner-Chef, Johnson's Supper Club, Elkader, Iowa, for all the information and recipes he supplied for this first revision.

Frances Nielsen, Oak Lawn, Illinois, who taught me so much of what I know about gourmet and ethnic cooking.

Vera and Aulden Wilson and Hazel and Ed Gernand, all of Wadena, Iowa, who spent so much time tasting and testing the recipes in this book and encouraging me to continue with it.

And finally, my husband, Chuck Cavaiani, and my sister, Shirley Sniffin. Their patience and support while I was writing this book have made it all possible.

I would also like to thank the following organizations for background information and resource material used in this book:
The American Diabetes Association, Inc.
The American Dietetic Association
The American Heart Association
Iowa State University Extension Service
U.S. Department of Agriculture
Iowa Affiliate of the American Diabetes Association

INTRODUCTION

This first revision of *The New Diabetic Cookbook* was written because the American Dietetic Association and The American Diabetes Association, Inc., prepared a new list of food exchanges for the diabetic diet in 1986. Not a great deal of revision was necessary, but there was enough to mandate a reassessment of the food exchanges of the recipes.

A great deal of study on the advantages of oat bran in the diabetic and low-cholesterol diets has also shown that we should take this matter very seriously and include recipes for the use of oat bran in this book. I have seen some remarkable results from the use of oat bran and am convinced that a substantial intake of oat bran will help lower both your glucose and cholesterol counts. We use it at our house every day, so I felt it was important to include information about and recipes for oat bran in the book, which reinforced our need for a first revision.

Once again I say, as I do in all of my special cookbooks: This is a cookbook, not a diet manual. Many books that are written to help people on a special diet are filled with "you can't do this" or "you must do that." I feel that no matter what your special diet may be, there are many familiar foods which you can and should have in your diet. Both Dr. Crockett and I feel that unless a diet includes familiar foods, it will not be followed, and that it is better to talk about the foods you are allowed rather than the ones which are no longer allowed on your diet.

I must admit that when I first became diabetic I felt as though the world had dropped out from under me. I remember telling my mother, "I'm such a good cook—and now I can't ever cook anything good again." That was a ridiculous statement, but it expressed my feelings at the time. It was a shock to me to discover that I was diabetic. We had always worried that my husband Chuck might become diabetic sometime because his mother, brother, sister, and nephew were all diagnosed as diabetic at different times—but we had never worried about me because no one in my family had diabetes.

I am a dietitian and should have recognized the symptoms, but I didn't. I only knew I felt terrible and didn't seem to get any better. I consulted Dr. Susan Urbatsch, my family doctor, who ordered a blood profile, and when the results were returned it was evident that I was diabetic. Of course, she investigated further but there wasn't much doubt about it after that first test.

I don't know if it is easier or harder for a diabetic who is also a dietitian. In one way it is easier because you don't need any diet counseling, you don't have questions regarding the suitability of different foods for your diet, and you don't have much trouble deciding if you can or can't have a certain food. However, I think it may actually be more difficult to be a dietitian because you are never free to relax and forget about your diet—you know what will happen to you if you do. I've seen too many people in the hospital or nursing home who were minus a foot or a leg or blind because they didn't think it made any difference whether they followed their diet and exercised regularly. It is so easy to say that you will put it off until tomorrow—but for a diabetic that tomorrow is right now and you'd better get with it or you will pay dearly for it later.

The low-cholesterol part of my diet didn't bother me because I had been keeping a low-cholesterol kitchen for many years. The doctor put my husband Chuck on a low-cholesterol diet when we were first married, and because I liked the diet and thought the food was good, I had always followed it right along with him. Dr. Urbatsch didn't tell me that I had a high cholesterol count or put me on a low-cholesterol diet, but the fact that 75 percent of all diabetics die of atherosclerosis or related diseases convinced me that I should follow a low-cholesterol diet even more carefully when I knew I was a diabetic.

All of the recipes in this book are suitable for a low-cholesterol diabetic diet. I might even suggest that if you are on a low-cholesterol diet and want to lose weight (even if you aren't a diabetic), you might find it useful to use these recipes to help take off those extra pounds. Fiber is included in many of these recipes because research has shown that fiber helps keep blood sugar lower for a diabetic and helps bring down the cholesterol count. Low-sodium variations are given for recipes whenever it is possible to prepare a low-sodium variation—I have found that so many people who need the low-cholesterol diabetic diet also have some sodium restrictions.

Our local diabetes association branch has been a big help to me. The support of others who have your problems seems to be particularly helpful, and this association is very active in providing information that is most useful to diabetics. I hope you will contact your own local association and let them help you as much as they have helped me.

I hope you will find these recipes helpful. I have tried to use foods that are nationally available and foods that most people stock regularly—I do dislike cookbooks that use recipes with strange-sounding names and even more unusual ingredients. These are recipes that my family and I use regularly and I hope they will become standards in your home also.

—Mabel Cavaiani, R.D.
Wadena, Iowa

THE
NEW
DIABETIC
C·O·O·K·B·O·O·K

1
FOOD EXCHANGES

Exchange lists are the backbone of the diabetic diet. The number and kind of exchanges you can use for each meal will be determined by your doctor and/or dietitian, depending upon your age, sex, amount of activity, and whether or not you need to lose weight. Each exchange has an established nutritional value. The total of your exchanges during the day is the total amount of carbohydrate, protein, and fat that your doctor determines you need to feel your best. Each of the exchanges contains foods that are of approximately the same nutritional value.

The following exchange lists (© 1986 American Diabetes Association, Inc., American Dietetic Association) have been reprinted with the permission of the American Diabetes Association and the American Dietetic Association. The exchange lists are the basis of a meal planning system designed by a committee of the American Diabetes Association and the American Dietetic Association. While designed primarily for people with diabetes and others who must follow special diets, the exchange lists are based on principles of good nutrition that apply to everyone. There are six basic exchanges with variations in some of the lists:

- **Starch/Bread exchanges** that contain 15 grams of carbohydrate, 3 grams of protein, a trace of fat, and 80 calories.

- **Meat exchanges** that are divided into 3 categories (values are for 1 ounce):

  Lean meat exchanges that contain 7 grams protein, 3 grams fat, and 55 calories.

  Medium-fat meat exchanges that contain 7 grams protein, 5 grams fat, and 75 calories.

  High-fat meat exchanges that contain 7 grams protein, 8 grams fat, and 100 calories.

- **Vegetable exchanges** that contain 5 grams of carbohydrate, 2 grams of protein, and 25 calories.

- **Fruit exchanges** that contain 15 grams carbohydrate and 60 calories.

- **Milk exchanges** that are divided into 3 categories (values are for 1 cup, or 8 ounces):

  Skim milk exchanges that contain 12 grams carbohydrate, 8 grams protein, trace of fat, and 90 calories.

  Low-fat milk exchanges that contain 12 grams carbohydrate, 8 grams protein, 5 grams fat, and 120 calories.

  Whole milk exchanges that contain 12 grams carbohydrate, 8 grams protein, 8 grams fat, and 150 calories.

- **Fat exchanges** that contain 5 grams of fat and 45 calories.

They are called exchanges because you can exchange one kind of food for another kind of food in the same exchange list using the quantities determined by the chart. This will provide for more variety in your diet without upsetting it.

Since you are concerned with the low-cholesterol diet as well as the diabetic diet, it is also important in your meal planning to consider which of the fats are saturated (animal fats), polyunsaturated (vegetable oils), or monosaturated (some vegetable oils). You want to avoid the saturated fats and emphasize the polyunsaturated fats. Monosaturated fats have been found to be more helpful than we realized. Since you are limited in the amount of fats that you can have, it is a good idea to concentrate on the polyunsaturated fats that help reduce cholesterol. Therefore it is important to use skim milk, egg whites instead of whole eggs, margarine instead of butter, and vegetable oil for cooking instead of lard or other animal fats such as butter.

Starch/bread items each contain approximately 15 grams of carbohydrate, 3 grams of protein, a trace of fat, and 80 calories. Whole-grain products average about 2 grams of fiber per serving. Foods that contain 3 or more grams of fiber are marked with an asterisk (*). You can choose your bread/starch exchanges from any of the items on the list. If you want to eat a starch food that is not on this list, the general rule is: ½ cup of cereal, grain, or pasta is 1 serving, and 1 ounce of a bread product is 1 serving. Your dietitian can help you be more exact.

Bread can be an excellent source of fiber, vitamin B, and potassium. Whole-wheat and bran breads, dried peas and beans, lentils, pumpkin, and squash are all excellent sources of fiber. The water-soluble dietary fiber in oat bran has proved to be particularly helpful in helping lower and/or control blood sugar and cholesterol in the blood.

Bread exchanges indicating 1 slice of bread refer to the size slice used by commercial bakers and not to homemade or fancy breads from the bakery. Refer to recipes in this book for low-cholesterol breads suitable for diabetics and use the portions given for those breads. Don't buy fancy breads in a bakery unless you know exactly what is used to make those breads. They are often high in sugar, and high in cholesterol from egg yolks or lard or other animal fats. If you have a bread recipe of your own that you want to use which doesn't contain any sugar or saturated fat, you can calculate it according to the information in Chapter 2 and then decide how many slices per loaf you need to equal 1 bread exchange per slice.

Some vegetables are included in the list of bread exchanges because they contain the same amount of carbohydrate and protein as 1 bread exchange.

Bread exchanges include the following:

½	1-ounce bagel
2	crisp bread sticks, 4 inches long by ½ inch wide (⅔ ounce each)
1 cup	low-fat croutons
½	English muffin
½	frankfurter or hamburger roll (1 ounce)

Cereals, Grains, Pasta

⅓ cup	bran cereals, concentrated cereals*
½ cup	flaked bran cereal (such as Bran Buds, All Bran, Fiber One)*
½ cup	cooked bulgur
½ cup	cooked cereals
2½ tablespoons	dry cornmeal
3 tablespoons	Grapenuts
½ cup	cooked grits
¾ cup	other ready-to-eat, unsweetened cereals

½ cup   cooked pasta
1½ cups   puffed cereals
⅓ cup   cooked white or brown rice
½ cup   shredded wheat
3 tablespoons   wheat germ*

Dried beans, peas, lentils

⅓ cup   cooked beans (such as kidney or white) and peas (such as split or black-eyed)*
⅓ cup   cooked lentils*
¼ cup   baked beans

Starchy vegetables

½ cup   corn*
1   6-inch ear corn on the cob*
½ cup   lima beans*
½ cup   green peas (canned or frozen)*
½ cup   plantain*
1   3-ounce baked potato*
½ cup   mashed potato
¾ cup   winter squash (acorn, butternut)
⅓ cup   plain yam or sweet potato

Starchy foods prepared with fat
(count as 1 starch bread serving plus 1 fat serving)

1   biscuit, 2½ inches across
½ cup   chow-mein noodles
1   2-inch cube corn bread (1½ ounces)
6   round, butter-type crackers
10   french-fried potatoes, 2 inches to 3½ inches long (1½ ounces)
1   plain, small muffin
2   4-inch pancakes
¼ cup   prepared bread stuffing
2   6-inch taco shells
1   4½-inch-square waffle
4–6   whole wheat crackers with fat added, such as Triscuits (1 ounce)
½   6-inch pita
1   1-ounce plain roll
1   1-ounce slice unfrosted raisin bread
1   1-ounce slice rye or pumpernickel bread*

1   6-inch tortilla
1   1-ounce slice white, French, or Italian bread
1   1-ounce slice whole wheat bread

Crackers, snacks

8   animal crackers
3   2½-inch-square graham crackers
¾ ounce   matzo
5 slices   melba toast
24   oyster crackers
3 cups   popcorn, popped without fat
¾ ounce   pretzels
4   Rye Krisp, 1 inches by 3½ inches
6   saltine-type crackers
2 to 4   whole wheat crackers without fat, such as Finn, Kavil, Wasa, (¾ ounce)*

Meats are our biggest problem when planning the low-cholesterol diabetic diet. It is comparatively easy to plan the meat exchanges. One meat exchange is 1 ounce cooked meat and it is a lean, medium-fat, or high-fat meat according to the charts. However, because of the low-cholesterol diet, it is best to stick to the lean meat list of the meat exchanges. The high-fat and even the medium-fat meats contain too much animal fat for a good low-cholesterol diet. (Read Chapter 10, Meats, for more detail about meat in the low-cholesterol diet.)

Some meats are high in sodium. Such meats are indicated by a double asterisk (**).

The American Dietetic Association and the American Diabetes Association, Inc., provide the following guidelines to help you keep the fat content of your diabetic diet at a manageable level.

1. Bake, roast, grill, or boil these meats rather than fry them with added fat.
2. Use a nonstick cooking spray or a nonstick pan to brown or fry these foods.
3. Trim off all visible fat before and after cooking.
4. Do not add flour, bread crumbs, coating mixes, or fat to these foods when preparing them.
5. Weigh meat after removing bones and fat and after cooking. Three ounces of cooked meat is about equal to 4 ounces of raw meat.

Some examples of meat portions are:

- 2 ounces meat (2 meat exchanges) are equal to 1 small chicken leg or thigh or ½ cup cottage cheese or tuna.
- 3 ounces meat (3 meat exchanges) are equal to 1 medium pork chop, 1 small hamburger, ½ of a whole chicken breast, 1 unbreaded fish fillet, or cooked meat about the size of a deck of cards.

6. If dried beans, peas, or lentils are used as a meat substitute, 1 cup of them cooked provides 3 grams or more of fiber and 2 starches and 1 lean meat exchanges.

Lean meat exchanges are for cooked weights and include the following:

Beef	USDA "Good" or "Choice" grades of lean beef, such as round, sirloin, or flank steak; tenderloin; or chipped beef.**
Pork	1 ounce lean pork, such as fresh ham, canned or cured or boiled ham**, Canadian bacon**, or tenderloin.
Veal	1 ounce of lean veal, such as chops or roasts. All cuts are lean except for ground or cubed veal cutlets.
Poultry	1 ounce chicken, turkey, or Cornish hen without skin.
Fish	1 ounce all fresh and frozen fish; 2 ounces crab, lobster, scallops, shrimp, or clams (fresh or canned in water); 6 medium oysters; ¼ cup tuna** (canned in water); 1 ounce herring (uncreamed or smoked); or 2 medium sardines (canned).
Wild Game	1 ounce venison, rabbit, and squirrel; 1 ounce pheasant, duck, or goose without skin.
Cheese	¼ cup any cottage cheese, 2 tablespoons grated Parmesan, or 1 ounce diet cheese** with less than 55 calories per ounce.
Other	1 ounce 95 percent fat-free luncheon meat, 3 egg whites, or ¾ cup egg substitutes with less than 55 calories per ¼ cup.

Vegetables are attractive, taste good, add bulk and fiber to the diet—and all this for very little carbohydrate. Vegetables do not contain any cholesterol and therefore you can use as many of them as you like within the diabetic diet. There are even some vegetables which you can eat as much of as you like, as long as they are raw. I hate to think how frustrated I would get on occasion if I couldn't satisfy my appetite between meals with carrot sticks and celery. My neighbor, Jan Franks, has a marvelous idea for parties. She puts out a big tray of fresh vegetables with a low-calorie dip. Anyone who is counting calories can munch on those and not worry about adding any exchanges to their diet that they will have to worry about later.

Vegetables are a good source of vitamins and minerals. Fresh and frozen vegetables have more vitamins and less salt than canned or prepared vegetables. Rinsing canned vegetables will remove much of the salt.

Vegetable exchanges, which are ½ cup cooked or 1 cup raw, contain about 5 grams of carbohydrate, 2 grams of protein, and 25 calories. Vegetables contain 2 to 3 grams of dietary fiber. Like meat, vegetables that contain 400 milligrams of sodium per serving are identified with a double asterisk (**). Starchy vegetables such as corn, peas, and potatoes are found on the starch/bread list.

Vegetable exchanges include the following:

Artichoke (½ medium)
Asparagus
Beans (green, wax, Italian)
Bean sprouts
Beets
Broccoli
Brussels sprouts
Cabbage, cooked
Carrots
Cauliflower
Eggplant
Greens (collard, mustard, turnip)
Kohlrabi
Leeks
Mushrooms, cooked
Okra
Onions
Pea pods
Green peppers
Rutabagas
Sauerkraut**
Spinach, cooked
Summer squash (crookneck)
Tomato (1 large)
Tomato/vegetable juice*
Turnips
Water chestnuts
Zucchini, cooked

Free vegetables contain less than 20 calories per serving. You can eat as much as you like of these raw vegetables without a specified serving size. Be sure to spread these out during the day. Vegetables with an asterisk (*) have 3 grams or more of dietary fiber per cup.

Cabbage
Celery
Chinese cabbage
Cucumber
Green onions
Hot peppers
Mushrooms
Radishes
Salad greens (endive, escarole, lettuce, romaine, spinach)
Zucchini*

Fruits may be used fresh, frozen, dried, or canned as long as no sugar is added. Fruits may be eaten as fresh fruit out of hand or in a salad or other combinations. I like to save my fruit exchanges for snacks, but many other people like to use them with their meals. Fruits add a great deal to our diets because they are tasty, high in vitamins and minerals, and a wonderful source of fiber. Several fruits are also a valuable source of potassium.

Fruit exchanges contain about 15 grams of carbohydrate and 60 calories. Fresh, frozen, and dry fruits have about 2 grams of fiber per serving. Fruits that have 3 grams or more of dietary fiber per serving have an asterisk (*). Fruit juices have very little dietary fiber. Unless otherwise noted, the serving size for a fruit exchange is ½ cup of fresh fruit or fruit juice or ¼ cup of dried fruit. Fruits do not contain cholesterol (except for coconut and coconut oil) and therefore may be used as desired within the framework of your diabetic diet.

Fruit exchanges include the following:

1	2-inch apple
½ cup	unsweetened applesauce
4	medium fresh apricots
½ cup or 4 halves	canned apricots
½	9-inch banana
¾ cup	fresh blackberries*
¾ cup	fresh blueberries*
⅓	5-inch cantaloupe
1 cup	cantaloupe cubes

12	large fresh cherries
½ cup	canned cherries
2	2-inch figs
½ cup	canned fruit cocktail
½	medium grapefruit
¾ cup	grapefruit segments
15	small grapes
⅛	medium honeydew melon
1 cup	honeydew melon cubes
1	large kiwi
¾ cup	mandarin orange slices
½	small mango
1	1½-inch nectarine*
1	2½-inch orange
1 cup	papaya
1	2¾-inch peach or ¾ cup peach slices
½ cup or 2 halves	canned peaches
½ large or 1 small	pear
½ cup or 2 halves	canned pears
2	medium native persimmons
¾ cup	raw pineapple
⅓ cup	canned pineapple
2	fresh 2-inch plums
½	pomegranate*
1 cup	fresh raspberries*
1¼ cups	fresh whole strawberries*
2	2½-inch tangerines
1¼ cups	watermelon cubes

Dried fruit

4 rings	apples
7 halves	apricots*
2½	medium dates
1½	figs*
3	medium prunes*
2 tablespoons	raisins

Fruit juice

½ cup	apple juice or cider
⅓ cup	cranberry juice cocktail

½ cup   grapefruit juice
⅓ cup   grape juice
½ cup   orange juice
½ cup   pineapple juice
⅓ cup   prune juice

A *free fruit* contains less than 20 calories per serving. You may eat 2 or 3 servings of these fruits per day. Be sure to spread the servings throughout the day.

½ cup   unsweetened cranberries
½ cup   unsweetened rhubarb

Milk is a good basic food in your meal plan because it is a good source of calcium, phosphorus, protein, and some of the B vitamins as well as vitamins A and D. I'm always upset when I hear someone say they don't like milk and never use it—I've seen so many older people with brittle bones that probably could have been prevented if they had used more milk in their diets earlier in their lives. If you don't want to drink milk, you can always use the instant dry milk in cooking or use yogurt or cheese in your meal plan. Cheese is a meat exchange, but it does provide calcium from the milk used to make the cheese, and you can add the vitamins to your diet with a good vitamin supplement. Even though you can't have most of the cheeses, you can always use low-fat cottage cheese, farmer's cheese, or ricotta—all of which are approved on a low-cholesterol diet.

Each serving of milk or milk products in the following table contains about 12 grams of carbohydrate and about 8 grams of protein. The amount of fat in milk is measured in percentage (%) of butterfat. The calories vary depending upon the kind of milk you use. People on a low-cholesterol diet should use either skim milk or nonfat dry milk for drinking and cooking. The table is divided into 3 parts based on the amount of fat and calories in one serving of skim/very low fat milk, low-fat milk, and whole milk.

NUTRITIVE VALUE OF DIFFERENT KINDS OF MILK

	Skim/Very low fat	Low-fat	Whole
Carbohydrate	12	12	12
Protein	8	8	8
Fat	Trace	5	8
Calories	90	120	150

Anyone on a low-cholesterol diet should use skim milk, low-fat yogurt, nonfat dry milk, or evaporated skim milk in order to avoid butterfat (the fat in the milk), which is a saturated fat.

Milk exchanges include the following:

1 cup	skim milk, ½% milk, 1% milk, low-fat buttermilk, or whole milk
8 ounces	plain low-fat yogurt with added nonfat milk solids or whole plain yogurt
½ cup	evaporated skim or whole milk
⅓ cup	nonfat dry milk

Fat exchanges should be used for unsaturated fats on a low-cholesterol diet. The following are 1 fat exchange of 5 grams fat and 45 calories. An asterisk (*) indicates that if more than 2 servings are eaten, the food will provide 400 or more milligrams of sodium.

Unsaturated fat exchanges include the following:

⅛	medium avocado
1 teaspoon	margarine or mayonnaise, or corn, cottonseed, safflower, soybean, olive, or peanut oils
1 tablespoon	diet margarine*, reduced-calorie mayonnaise*, dry-roasted cashews* or other nuts, seeds, pine nuts, sunflower oil, soybean oil, sunflower seeds without shells, or all varieties of salad dressing
2	whole walnuts, pecans
2 teaspoons	pumpkin seeds
20 small or 10 large	peanuts
10 small or 5 large	olives*
2 teaspoons	mayonnaise-type salad dressing
2 tablespoons	reduced-calorie salad dressing*
Up to 2 tablespoons	low-calorie salad dressing is a free food

Saturated fat exchanges

1 teaspoon	butter
1 slice	bacon*
2 tablespoons	shredded coconut, liquid coffee whitener, cream (light, coffee, table), sour cream
1 tablespoon	heavy whipping cream, cream cheese
4 teaspoons	powdered coffee whitener
¼ ounce	salt pork

And last but not least we come to that delightful group of foods known as **free foods**, which are foods that we can use without counting them as a food exchange. In some cases the amount is limited because too much of them would be a food exchange—but some of them can be used as desired.

Free sweet substitutes include hard, sugar-free candy; sugar-free gelatin; sugar-free gum; 2 teaspoons sugar-free jam or jelly; 1 to 2 tablespoons sugar-free pancake syrup; 2 tablespoons whipped topping; and sugar substitutes, such as aspartame (Equal) and saccharin.

Free condiments include 1 tablespoon catsup; 2 tablespoons low-calorie salad dressing; 1 tablespoon taco sauce, horseradish, and mustard; dill pickles; and vinegar.

Seasonings make food taste better. Be careful how much sodium you use. Read labels and choose seasonings that do not contain sodium or salt.

If you are limited in your sodium intake use low-sodium soy sauce instead of regular.

Up to ¼ cup wine is free when used as an ingredient in a recipe.

Spices, herbs, and flavorings as well as chives, celery, seed, hot-pepper sauce, lemon juice, lime juice, onion or garlic powder, pimiento, soy sauce, and Worcestershire are free foods.

2
CALCULATING FOOD EXCHANGES

Information about food exchanges is basic to good management of your diabetic diet. You need to learn as much about them as possible—what they are and how to use them.

Food exchanges are a method of measuring food values so that a diabetic can control the amount of carbohydrate and other nutrients consumed. The nutritional value of the exchanges has been determined by the American Dietetic Association. You can't change their values, but you can work with them better when you understand more about them. They have been standardized as follows:

The exchanges are established in grams—which are more familiar to other nationalities than to Americans since we are still using the British system of pounds and ounces. Grams are a measure of weight used in most laboratories and research centers here in our country as well as abroad. One ounce equals 28.35 grams, so that a 1-ounce slice of bread that contains 15 grams of carbohydrate is about half carbohydrate and the rest water, fiber, fat, and other ingredients. A vegetable exchange that weighs 3½ to 4 ounces contains only 5 grams of carbohydrate and therefore has a much smaller percentage of carbohydrate and a larger percentage of fiber, water, and other nutrients. A fruit exchange has about ½ ounce of carbohydrate, and a milk exchange has ⅓ to ½ ounce of carbohydrate in 8 ounces of milk. Since the percentage of carbohydrate in a food is important to us, it is helpful to realize that most vegetables have a much smaller percentage of carbohydrate than bread and some of the starchier vegetables.

COMPOSITION OF FOOD GROUPS OR EXCHANGES PER SERVING

Food Exchange	Carbohydrate (Gms.)	Protein (Gms.)	Fat (Gms.)	Calories
Starch/bread	15	3	Trace	80
Meat: Lean		7	3	55
Medium fat		7	5	75
High fat		7	8	100
Vegetable	5	2		25
Fruit	15			60
Milk: Skim, very low fat	12	8	Trace	90
Low fat	12	8	5	120
Whole	12	8	8	150
Fat			5	45

At first most diabetics tend to use recipes that have been calculated by someone else—it's hard enough to get used to thinking in terms of exchanges without worrying about how they were determined. After awhile, though, you begin to wonder why you can't use some of your own recipes. The next step generally is comparing a recipe that has been calculated with one of your own recipes and accepting the exchanges determined for the other recipe for your own recipe. This isn't too bad an idea, but it can cause trouble sometimes because the recipes aren't exactly alike. Some little ingredient in your recipe can throw the whole calculation off and your recipe may be less accurate than you realize.

The final and best step is learning to calculate your own recipes. Sometimes you may have to juggle your own around a bit—cutting out some of the flour, cutting down on the sugar, or substituting a low-carbohydrate vegetable for a high-starch one—but eventually you'll learn how to manage your own recipes after you learn to calculate them.

In order to establish the nutritive values of each portion in a recipe, you must calculate the total nutritive values of the complete recipe, divide by the number of servings the recipe yields, and then compare the nutritive values of each portion with the chart showing the carbohydrate, protein, and fat values of each of the exchanges.

Calculating your own recipes would be very difficult if it weren't for all of the excellent information available to us—thanks to so many dedicated people who have worked hard establishing the nutritive values of foods.

It is helpful to collect information about the nutritive values of foods you use every day. There is an increasing amount of help available from many sources. Now that most cans and packages include nutritive information on the labels, you can collect that information and use it to establish a file of your own. Many of the cereal companies have very complete information available regarding their products, and most companies will send it to you if you are unable to find it on the package. The following books contain information that is invaluable when calculating recipes:

Nutritive Value of American Foods in Common Units, Agricultural Handbook 456, U.S. Department of Agriculture. Washington, D.C.: Superintendent of Documents, U.S. Printing Office, 1975. $5.15

Nutritive Value of Foods, Home and Garden Bulletin 72, U.S. Department of Agriculture. Washington, D.C.: Superintendent of Documents, U.S. Printing Office, 1977.

Composition of Foods, Raw, Processed, and Prepared, Agriculture Handbook No. 8, U.S. Department of Agriculture. Washington, D.C.: Superintendent of Documents, U.S. Printing Office, 1963, and all current revisions.

Nutritive Value of Convenience Foods, published by West Suburban Dietetic Association (Laura Wilford, Editor, P.O. Box 1103, Hines, Illinois 60141), 1976. $9.00

Food Values of Portions Commonly Used, Bowes and Church, J. B. Lippincott Company.

The first three books are available in many large cities from the U.S. Government printing office stores, or may be ordered at your local county extension agent office or purchased from the Superintendent of Documents, U.S. Government Printing Office, Washington, D.C. 20402.

RECIPE ANALYSIS

The nutritive values that concern us most are calories (CAL), carbohydrate (CHO), protein (PRO), fat, and for some of us, sodium (NA). To calculate a recipe, the simplest procedure is to make a chart showing the list of ingredients and the nutritive values of each. When I started this book, I

RECIPE ANALYSIS

Name of recipe _____ Date tested _____

Source of recipe _____

Type and number of pans used _____

_____

Temperature _____ Number of servings _____

Baking or cooking time _____

Comments on recipe _____

Ingredient	Amount	Calories	CHO (gm)	PRO (gm)	Fat (gm)	NA (mg)
Total nutritive values						
Divided by the total number of portions						
Rounded to the nearest number						
Number of food exchanges equal to nutritive value:						

worked out the following form and took it to the printer so that I wouldn't have to draw it up every time I wanted to calculate a recipe. If you'd like, you can copy it for your own use, or you can draw up your own form to include whatever information you would like to have on the recipe. I didn't include cholesterol on the form; however, there is a table of cholesterol in the ingredients chapter, if you would like to check your cholesterol intake. Personally, I feel that you should avoid anything that contains cholesterol. Some dietitians and doctors tell you that you can have 2 or 3 eggs weekly; however, I feel that you should avoid egg yolks and other cholesterol-rich foods completely—at least when you are first starting your low-cholesterol diet and trying hard to bring down that cholesterol count.

When I use this form, I list the ingredients for each recipe and then look for the appropriate values for each ingredient in one of my references—for instance, as I did on page 18 for the cornbread recipe on page 249.

After you have calculated the total nutritive values of the recipe, divide the total of each of the elements (CAL, CHO, PRO, FAT, and NA) by the total number of portions to get the nutritive values per serving. Then compare it with the table at the beginning of this chapter to decide how many food exchanges you will get from each serving—as I did at the bottom of the recipe analysis.

ADJUSTING YOUR RECIPE

Your recipe probably won't turn out exactly the way you want it to the first time. I have tested most of the recipes in this book several times. The first time I test a recipe, I use the ingredients listed in the basic recipe, cutting down on the sugar or fat or whatever else I think I need to reduce. While some recipes need a little sugar for color and texture, you will be surprised at the amount of sugar you can take out of a recipe and still get a pretty good product. On the first test of a recipe with the sugar reduced, I add sugar substitute equal to the amount of sugar that I removed. I probably will cut down on the sugar substitute on the next testing because I don't like the taste of an excessive amount of it, but I need to determine how much I want to use in the final recipe. Remember when you are adding sugar substitute that Equal (NutraSweet) breaks down if it is baked or heated too long; if you are using prolonged heat, use some other kind of sugar substitute. I try to add Equal after I have taken whatever I'm cooking off the heat, which seems to work very well; or else I use it in things that don't need to be cooked, such as gelatin or fruit.

RECIPE ANALYSIS

Name of recipe _Yankee Cornbread_ Date tested _July 25_

Source of recipe _My favorite recipe_

Type and number of pans used _mixer bowl and 9-inch square baking pan_

Temperature _400 degrees_ Number of servings _16_

Baking or cooking time _25 minutes_

Comments on recipe _Chuck's favorite, good texture + color_

Ingredient	Amount	Calories	CHO (gm)	PRO (gm)	Fat (gm)	NA (mg)
cornmeal	1 cup	502	108.2	10.9	1.7	1
all-purpose flour	1 cup	455	95.1	13.1	1.3	3
baking powder	4 tsp	16	3.6	—	—	1,316
sugar	1/4 cup	193	49.8	—	—	tr
instant dry milk	1/4 cup	88	6.7	4.6	4.8	71
salt	1/4 tsp	—	—	—	—	533
liquid egg sub.	1/4 cup	30	1.0	6.0	—	90
vegetable oil	1/4 cup	482	—	—	54.5	—
Total nutritive values		1,766	264.4	34.6	62.3	2,014
Divided by the total number of portions (16)		110.4	16.53	2.16	3.89	125.88
Rounded to the nearest number		110	17	2	4	126
Number of food exchanges equal to nutritive value:						
1 bread			15	2		
1 fat					5	
total			15	2	5	

You can also reduce the fat in a recipe quite a bit, although you do need some fat in baked goods for texture and tenderness.

After the first time you test a recipe and calculate its nutritive values, you can decide how much more you need to cut ingredients in order to have a product suitable for your use. Sometimes the calories or fat or carbohydrate are too high and you need to try it again, cutting down on the offending ingredient. It is possible to repeatedly try a recipe and never get it right, but generally, you can work with it and find a variation of the original recipe that you can use. One important thing to remember is to write down exactly what you use when you are testing a recipe. It is so frustrating to get just what you want in a recipe and then forget exactly how much of each ingredient you used.

Another way to control the food exchanges is by dividing a recipe into the size portions that conform to what you can have. In the bread chapter, you will notice that the number of slices per loaf varies according to the recipe. That is because I need to cut a certain size slice to arrive at a bread exchange for each slice. To find this, I divide the total grams of carbohydrate in the recipe by 15, which is the amount allowed for a bread exchange; that tells me how many slices I need from each loaf in order to have each slice equal one bread exchange.

I find a calculator a big help when calculating recipes. It is much faster and gives me more confidence that my totals are correct.

When I became diabetic and had to calculate all my recipes, I realized how lucky I had been to work for Miriam H. Thomas back when I first started working for the government. Then a research chemist in Chicago, she introduced me to the world of food analysis and calculations. I remember telling her that I was a dietitian used to working in restaurants, and that I'd never get all of those calculations straight. She told me I was perfect for the job because a dietitian would realize the importance of calculating the nutritive values of the Army rations very carefully. So I persevered and eventually it all made sense.

After Miriam's office moved to Natick, Massachusetts, I worked for a few months for Mary Klicka, a dietitian/nutritionist at the same center. Among other things, Mary was developing foods for the space program and I learned something new and interesting every day. She used to fascinate me with her knowledge of the nutritive content of almost anything, and has given me the nutritive analysis of several foods that I couldn't find in any of my other references.

After Mary Klicka moved to Natick, I transferred to the Menu Planning Division of the Army Food Service Center in Chicago, where I worked for several years under the direction of Marion Bollman. While there, I worked on Army menus and also learned how to write recipes. When the Armed Forces decided to set up a joint recipe file, Marion appointed me as the Army representative on the Armed Forces Recipe Service File Committee. We spent a lot of time working on that file, which was a real learning experience and gave me the background necessary to start writing my own cookbooks.

As an aid in developing recipes for my cookbooks, I keep a chart of nutritive values of many ingredients that I use a lot so I don't have to look them up every time. This is very helpful to me, and since it is likely to be helpful for you also, I'm including it in this chapter. I have only included foods which may be used on a low-cholesterol diet. I have not included egg yolks, cream, or other high-fat foods. However, I did relent and include chocolate chips because you might like to use them occasionally—and you should have their nutritive value so you will know how many you can use.

When calculating meat recipes, I subtract the values for any fat that cooks out of the meat, using the values for fat in the chart. I chill the fat and then measure it very carefully after it is hardened in the refrigerator.

Although you can't use much of them, I have included sugars because research now shows a little can be used as long as it is calculated in the total exchanges for that food. You might discuss this with your doctor; however, most doctors and dietitians concur that a small amount will not upset your sugar count.

The following measures may also help you in your calculations:

3 teaspoons = 1 tablespoon
4 tablespoons = ¼ cup
5⅓ tablespoons = ⅓ cup
8 tablespoons = ½ cup
10⅔ tablespoons = ⅔ cup
12 tablespoons = ¾ cup
16 tablespoons = 1 cup
2 cups = 1 pint
4 cups = 1 quart
4 quarts = 1 gallon
16 ounces = 1 pound

I have used pound and cup measures for many items in this table so that from them you can calculate your own recipes.

Remember as you are using this information that it is specifically aimed at the person on a low-cholesterol diabetic diet. All values for fruits and fruit juices are without any added sweetener and meats which are high in fat are not included—nor are any other products which are not approved on a low-cholesterol diet.

I hope you will be encouraged to use this information in calculating your own favorite recipes and to devise variations of other recipes which will help to add some spice and variety to your diet.

NUTRIENT ANALYSIS OF MEATS

	Amount	Calories	CHO (gm)	PRO (gm)	Fat (gm)	NA (mg)
BEEF						
Chuck, raw, good grade, without fat or bone	1 lb.	739		96.2	36.3	
Dried Beef	1 lb.	921		155.6	28.6	19,509
Flank Steak, raw, good grade	1 lb.	631		98.9	23.1	
Hamburger						
raw, 10% fat	1 lb.	812		93.9	45.4	
cooked, 10% fat	1 lb.	995		124.4	51.3	218
raw, 20% fat	1 lb.	1,216		81.2	96.2	
cooked, 20%	1 lb.	1,298		109.9	92.2	213
Round, raw, choice, without fat or bone	1 lb.	612		98.0	21.3	
Rump						
raw, good grade, without fat or bone	1 lb.	640		98.0	24.5	
cooked	1 lb.	863		134.4	32.2	
Sirloin Steak						
raw, good grade, without fat or bone	1 lb.	585		98.9	18.1	
cooked	1 lb.	830		143.9	24.1	
LAMB						
Loin chops, raw, without fat cut 4 to the pound	1 chop	92		13.8	3.7	34

Leg

raw, without bone	1 lb.	1,007	80.7	73.5	282
	1 oz.	63	5.0	4.6	18
cooked, without fat or bone	1 lb.	844	130.2	31.8	319
	1 oz.	53	8.1	2.0	20
Shoulder, raw, lean without fat	1 lb.	930	121.6	45.4	298
	1 oz.	58	7.6	2.8	19

PORK

Loin, raw, without fat or bone	1 lb.	857	91.2	51.7	1,453
	1 oz.	54	5.7	3.2	91
Fresh pork ham, without fat or bone	1 lb.	694	90.7	34.0	1,453
	1 oz.	44	5.7	2.1	91

Ham

raw, without fat, bone, or skin	1 lb.	1,209	76.1	98.0	3,896
	1 oz.	76	4.8	6.1	244
cooked, without fat, bone, or skin	1 lb.	848	114.8	39.9	4,110
	1 oz.	53	7.2	2.5	257

VEAL

Round, raw, without bone	1 lb.	744	88.5	41.0	320
	1 oz.	47	5.5	2.6	20
Loin, raw, without bone	1 lb.	821	87.1	50.0	320
	1 oz.	51	5.4	3.1	20
Cooked, chopped	1 cup	328	37.0	18.8	91

NUTRIENT ANALYSIS OF POULTRY

	Amount	Calories	CHO (gm)	PRO (gm)	Fat (gm)	NA (mg)
CHICKEN						
Broiler-fryer, without skin	2½ lb. chicken	480		84.0	13.4	232
Raw, without fat, bones, or skin, average of light and dark meat	1 lb.	776		135.2	22.0	340
	1 oz.	49		8.5	1.4	21
Roast, cooked, without fat, bones, or skin, average of light and dark meat	1 lb.	831		139.7	25.9	304
	1 oz.	52		8.7	1.6	19
Chopped, cooked, without fat, bones, or skin, average of light and dark meat	1 cup	239		41.7	6.9	105
TURKEY						
Cooked, without fat, bones, or skin, average of light and dark meat	1 cup	266		44.1	8.5	182
	1 oz.	54		8.9	1.7	37

NUTRIENT ANALYSIS OF FISH

	Amount	Calories	CHO (gm)	PRO (gm)	Fat (gm)	NA (mg)
FISH						
Catfish, fillets, raw	1 lb.	467		79.8	14.1	272
Codfish, raw	1 lb.	354		79.8	1.4	318
Flounder and sole, raw	1 lb.	358		75.8	3.6	354
Haddock, raw	1 lb.	358		83.0	.5	277
Halibut, raw	1 lb.	454		94.8	5.4	245
Mackerel, raw,						
Atlantic	1 lb.	866		86.2	55.3	
Pacific	1 lb.	721		99.3	33.1	
Perch, white, raw	1 lb.	535		87.5	18.1	
Perch, yellow, raw	1 lb.	413		88.5	4.1	308
Pike, northern, raw	1 lb.	399		83.0	5.0	
Pike, walleye, raw	1 lb.	422		87.5	6.4	231
Red and gray snapper, raw	1 lb.	422		89.8	4.1	304
Salmon, fresh	1 lb.	984		102.1	60.8	
Salmon, canned, red	1 lb.	776		92.1	42.2	2,368
Salmon, canned, pink	1 lb.	640		93.0	26.8	1,755
Swordfish, raw	1 lb.	535		87.1	18.1	
Tuna, raw, bluefin	1 lb.	658		114.3	18.6	
Tuna, canned, in water	6½ oz.	234		51.5	1.5	75
Whiting, raw	1 lb.	476		83.0	13.6	376
Whitefish, raw	1 lb.	703		85.7	37.2	236

NUTRIENT ANALYSIS OF CEREALS AND STARCHES

	Amount	Calories	CHO (gm)	PRO (gm)	Fat (gm)	NA (mg)
Barley, pearl, light	1 cup	698	157.6	16.4	2.0	6
Bran, wheat	1 cup	144	44.6	7.6	1.8	493
Breads, commercial						
French or Vienna	1 oz slice	82	15.7	2.6	.9	164
rye	1 oz slice	61	13.0	2.3	.3	139
white	1 oz slice	78	14.2	2.6	1.1	140
whole wheat	1 oz slice	69	13.5	3.0	.9	149
Bread crumbs, dry	1 cup	392	73.4	12.6	4.6	736
Bulgur, dry, cracked wheat	1 cup	628	139.1	15.2	2.5	1
Cornmeal	1 cup	502	108.2	10.9	1.7	1
Cornstarch	1 tbsp	29	7.0	tr	tr	tr
Flour						
all-purpose	1 cup	455	95.1	13.1	1.3	3
bread	1 cup	499	104.3	14.4	1.4	3
cake	1 cup	430	93.7	8.9	.9	2
rye, light	1 cup	364	79.5	9.6	1.0	1
soybean, low-fat	1 cup	313	32.2	38.2	5.9	1
whole wheat or graham	1 cup	400	85.2	16.0	2.4	4
Graham crackers	1 double	55	10.4	1.1	1.3	95
crumbs	1 cup	326	62.3	6.8	8.0	570

Food	Measure					
Macaroni, dry	1 lb	1,674	341.1	56.7	5.4	9
cooked	1 cup	155	32.2	4.8	.6	1
Noodles, dry, commercial	1 lb	1,760	326.6	58.1	20.9	23
cooked	1 cup	200	37.3	6.6	2.4	3
chow mein	1 cup	220	26.1	5.9	10.6	
Oat bran	1 cup	217	64.8	17.1	4.0	23
Rice						
brown, raw	1 cup	666	143.2	13.9	3.5	17
brown, cooked	1 cup	173	37.0	3.6	.9	409
white, instant, dry	1 cup	355	78.4	7.1	.2	1
white, long-grain, raw	1 cup	672	148.7	12.4	.7	9
white, long-grain, cooked	1 cup	158	35.1	2.9	.1	767
wild, raw	1 cup	565	120.5	22.6	1.1	11
Rolled oats, dry	1 cup	312	54.6	11.4	5.9	2
Rolled wheat, dry	1 cup	289	64.8	8.4	17	2
Sesame seed	1 tbsp	47	1.4	1.5	4.3	
Tapioca, dry, pearl	1 tbsp	30	7.3	.1	tr	tr

NUTRIENT ANALYSIS OF SUGARS

	Amount	Calories	CHO (gm)	PRO (gm)	Fat (gm)	NA (mg)
Chocolate chips, semisweet	1 cup	862	96.9	7.1	60.7	3
	1 tbsp	54	6.1	.4	3.8	tr
Equal (Nutrasweet)	1 pkt	4	.96			
Honey	1 cup	1,031	279.0	1.0		17
	1 tbsp	64	17.4	.1		1
Molasses, dark	1 cup	699	180.4			315
	1 tbsp	44	11.3			20
Sugar, brown	1 cup	821	212.1			66
	1 tbsp	51	13.3			4
Sugar, powdered	1 cup	385	100			1
	1 tbsp	24	6			tr
Sugar, granulated	1 cup	770	199.0			
	1 tbsp	48	12.4			
Syrup, maple	1 cup	794	204.8			32
	1 tbsp	50	12.8			2
Syrup, sorghum	1 cup	848	224.4			
	1 tbsp	53	14.0			
Syrup, corn	1 cup	951	246.0			223
	1 tbsp	59	15.4			14
Syrup, cane and maple	1 cup	794	204.8			6
	1 tbsp	50	12.8			tr

NUTRIENT ANALYSIS OF FATS AND NUTS

	Amount	Calories	CHO (gm)	PRO (gm)	Fat (gm)	NA (mg)
FATS						
Margarine	1 stick-½ cup	816	.5	.7	91.9	1,119
	1 tbsp	102	.1	.1	11.5	140
Vegetable oil	1 cup	1,927			218.0	
	1 tbsp	120			13.6	
NUTS						
Almonds, shelled	1 lb	2,713	88.5	84.4	245.9	18
chopped	1 cup	777	25.4	24.2	70.5	5
Cashews, roasted, in oil	1 lb	2,545	132.9	78.0	207.3	68
	1 cup	785	41.0	24.1	64.0	21
Peanuts, roasted, whole	1 lb	2,654	85.3	117.9	225.9	1,896
chopped	1 cup	842	27.1	37.4	7.7	602
Pecans, roasted, whole	1 lb	3,116	66.2	41.7	323.0	tr
	1 cup	811	17.2	10.9	84.0	tr
Walnuts, English, roasted, whole	1 lb	2,953	71.7	67.1	290.3	9
chopped	1 cup	781	19.0	17.8	76.8	2
Average of nuts used in this book	1 lb	2,796	88.9	77.8	258.5	398
	1 cup	799	25.9	22.9	73.4	126
Peanut butter	1 cup	1,520	48.5	65.0	130.5	1,561
	1 tbsp	95	3	4	8.2	98

NUTRIENT ANALYSIS OF DAIRY PRODUCTS AND EGGS

	Amount	Calories	CHO (gm)	PRO (gm)	Fat (gm)	NA (mg)
Egg white, large	1	17	.3	3.6	tr	48
Egg substitute, liquid	1 cup	120	4.0	24.0		360
	¼ cup	30	1.0	6.0		90
Cheese						
cottage, large curd, with 4% milk	1 cup	239	6.5	30.6	9.5	515
small curd, with 4% milk	1 cup	223	6.1	28.6	8.8	481
packed dry	1 cup	172	5.4	34.0	.6	580
mozzarella, made from part skim milk	1 oz.	80	1.0	8.0	5.0	not available
Parmesan, grated	1 tbsp	23	.2	2.1	1.5	44
ricotta, made with part skim milk	1 cup	340	13.0	28.0	19.0	not available
Ice milk, hard	1 cup	199	29.3	6.3	6.7	255
soft serve	1 cup	266	29.3	8.4	8.9	89
Milk						
dry buttermilk	1 cup	464	60.0	41.2	6.4	608
	1 tbsp	29	3.8	2.6	.4	38
skim fresh	1 cup	88	12.5	8.8	.2	127
evaporated	1 cup	200	29.0	19.0	1.0	254

instant dry, nonfat	1 cup	224	35.5	23.9	.5	373
	1 tbsp	15	2.2	1.5	.2	23
	⅓ cup	81	11.8	8.0		124
Yogurt (nonfat)						
plain	8 oz	125	17.0	13.0	t	125
fruit flavored	8 oz	230	42.0	10.0	3.0	125

NUTRIENT ANALYSIS OF FRUITS AND VEGETABLES
(All Fruits and Fruit juices are unsweetened)

	Amount	Calories	CHO (gm)	PRO (gm)	Fat (gm)	NA (mg)
Apricots, raw	1 lb	217	54.6	4.3	.9	4
canned	1 cup	93	23.6	1.7	.2	2
Apples, fresh	1 (¼ lb)	61	15.3	.2	.6	1
Applesauce, canned	1 cup	100	26.4	.5	.5	5
Asparagus, raw	1 lb.	118	22.7	11.3	.9	9
cooked, cuts	1 cup	29	5.2	3.2	.3	1
canned, cuts	1 cup	52	8.5	4.9	1.2	555
Avocado	1 avg (10-11 oz)	378	14.3	4.8	37.1	9
Banana, whole	1 med	101	26.4	1.3	.2	1
mashed	1 cup	191	50.0	2.5	.5	2
Beans, dry, great northern	1 cup	612	110.3	40.1	2.9	34
cooked	1 cup	212	38.2	14.0	1.1	13
Beans, dry, kidney	1 cup	635	114.5	41.6	2.8	19
cooked	1 cup	218	39.6	14.4	.9	6
Beans, lima, dry	1 cup	621	115.2	36.7	2.9	7
cooked	1 cup	262	48.6	15.6	1.1	4
Beans, lima, green, cooked	1 cup	189	33.7	12.9	.9	2
Beans, green, raw	1 cup	35	7.8	2.1	.2	8
cooked	1 cup	31	6.8	2.0	.3	5
canned	1 cup	43	10.0	2.4	.2	564
frozen	1 cup	33	7.5	2.1	.1	1

Beans, wax, raw	1 cup	30	6.6	1.9	.2	8
cooked	1 cup	28	5.8	1.8	.3	4
canned	1 cup	45	10.0	2.4	.5	564
Bean sprouts, mung, cooked	1 cup	35	6.5	4.0	.3	5
Beets, raw, diced	1 cup	58	13.4	2.2	.1	81
cooked, diced	1 cup	54	12.2	1.9	.2	73
canned	1 cup	84	19.4	2.2	.2	581
Blackberries, or boysenberries, raw	1 cup	84	18.6	1.7	1.3	1
canned	1 cup	98	22.0	2.0	1.5	2
Blueberries, raw	1 cup	90	22.2	1.0	.7	1
frozen	1 cup	91	22.4	1.2	.8	2
Broccoli, raw	1 lb	145	26.8	16.3	1.4	68
cooked, stems and pieces	1 cup	40	7.0	4.8	.5	16
frozen, chopped	1 lb	132	23.6	14.5	1.4	77
frozen, cooked	10 oz pkg	65	11.5	7.3	.8	38
Brussels sprouts, raw	1 lb	204	37.6	22.2	1.8	64
cooked	1 cup	56	9.9	6.5	.6	16
Cabbage, raw	1 lb	109	24.5	5.9	.9	91
shredded, raw	1 cup	17	3.8	.9	.1	14
cooked	1 cup	29	6.2	1.6	.3	20
Celery cabbage, raw	1 lb	64	13.6	5.4	.5	104
	1 cup	11	2.0	1.1	.1	18
cooked	1 cup	24	4.1	2.4	.3	31
Carrots, raw, no tops	1 lb	191	44	5.0	.9	213
shredded, raw	1 cup	46	10.7	1.2	.2	52
cooked	1 cup	48	11.0	1.4	.3	51

NUTRIENT ANALYSIS OF FRUITS AND VEGETABLES (Cont.)

	Amount	Calories	CHO (gm)	PRO (gm)	Fat (gm)	NA (mg)
Cauliflower, raw	1 lb	122	23.6	12.2	.9	59
cooked	1 cup	28	5.1	2.9	.3	11
frozen	10-oz pkg	62	12.2	5.7	.6	31
Celery, raw	1 lb	77	17.7	4.1	.5	572
diced or chopped, raw	1 cup	20	4.7	1.1	.1	151
diced, cooked	1 cup	21	4.7	1.2	.2	132
Cherries, raw, whole, red sour	1 cup	60	14.7	1.2	.3	2
whole, sweet, raw	1 cup	82	20.4	1.5	.4	2
canned, red	1 cup	105	26.1	2.0	.5	5
canned, sweet	1 cup	119	29.6	2.2	.5	2
candied	1 oz	96	24.6	.1	.1	
Chives, raw	1 tbsp	1	.2	.1	tr	
Collard greens, raw, leaves and stems	1 lb	181	32.7	16.3	3.2	195
frozen, chopped	1 lb	145	26.3	14.1	1.8	82
cooked	1 cup	51	9.5	4.9	.7	27
Sweet corn, raw, whole kernels	1 lb	240	55.1	8.7	2.5	tr
cooked	1 cup	137	31.0	5.3	1.7	tr
canned	1 cup	174	43.1	5.3	1.1	496
frozen	10-oz pkg	233	55.9	8.8	1.4	3
Cream style corn, canned	1 cup	210	51.2	5.4	1.5	604
Cowpeas or blackeye, dry	1 cup	583	104.9	38.8	2.6	60
cooked	1 cup	190	34.5	12.8	.8	20
Cranberries, raw	1 lb	200	47.0	1.7	3.0	9
	1 cup	44	10.3	.4	.7	2

Cucumbers, raw, pared	1 lb	68	15.4	4.1	.5	27
sliced	1 cup	16	3.6	.9	.1	6
Dates, pitted	1 lb.	1,243	330.7	10.0	2.3	5
	1 cup	488	129.8	3.9	.9	2
Dill pickles, sliced	1 cup	17	3.4	1.1	.3	2,213
Eggplant, diced, cooked	1 cup	38	8.2	2.0	.4	2
Endive or Escarole, raw	1 lb	91	18.6	7.7	.5	64
chopped	1 cup	10	2.1	.9	.1	7
Figs, raw, whole	1 med	40	10.2	.6	.2	1
canned	1 cup	119	30.8	1.2	.5	5
Fruit cocktail, canned	16-oz can	168	44.0	1.8	.5	23
	1 cup	91	23.8	1.0	.2	12
Garlic, clove	1	4	.9	.2	tr	1
Ginger, root, fresh	1 lb	207	40.1	5.9	4.2	25
Gooseberries, raw	1 cup	59	14.6	1.2	3	2
Grapefruit, pink, raw	½	40	10.3	.5	1	1
Grapefruit, white, raw	½	56	14.7	.7	1	1
seedless	½	46	11.9	.6	1	1
canned	1 cup	73	18.5	1.5	2	10
Grapes:						
Concord	1 lb	207	47.0	3.9	3.0	9
seedless	1 lb	107	27.7	1.0	.5	5
Tokay	1 lb	102	26.3	.9	.5	5
Guava	1 lb	273	66.0	3.5	2.6	18

NUTRIENT ANALYSIS OF FRUITS AND VEGETABLES (Cont.)

	Amount	Calories	CHO (gm)	PRO (gm)	Fat (gm)	NA (mg)
Kale, raw	1 lb	240	40.8	27.2	3.6	340
cooked	1 cup	40	7.0	3.9	.7	27
frozen	10-oz pkg	91	15.6	9.1	1.4	74
Kohlrabi, raw	1 cup	41	9.2	2.8	.1	11
Lemon, raw	1 med	20	6.0	.8	.2	1
juice	1 tbsp	4	1.2	.1	tr	tr
Lettuce	1 lb	59	13.2	4.1	.5	41
chopped	1 cup	7	1.6	.5	.1	5
Lime, raw	1	19	6.4	.5	.1	1
juice	1 tbsp	4	1.4	tr	tr	tr
Mandarin oranges	1 cup	90	22.6	1.6	.4	4
Mango, raw	1 lb	299	76.2	3.2	1.8	32
Mushrooms, raw	1 lb	127	20.0	12.2	1.4	68
chopped	1 cup	20	3.1	1.9	.2	11
canned	4-oz can	17	2.4	1.9	.1	400
Muskmelon, cubed or diced						
cantaloupe	1 cup	48	12.0	1.1	.2	19
casaba	1 cup	46	11.1	2.0	tr	20
honeydew	1 cup	56	13.1	1.4	.5	20
Mustard greens, raw	1 lb.	141	25.4	13.6	2.3	145
cooked	1 cup	32	5.6	3.1	.6	25
frozen	10 oz pkg	57	9.1	6.5	1.1	34
Nectarine	1	88	23.6	.8	tr	8
Okra, raw	1 lb	163	34.5	10.9	1.4	14
cooked	1 cup	46	9.6	3.2	.5	3
frozen	10-oz pkg	111	25.6	6.5	.3	6

Onions, dry	1 lb	172	39.5	6.8	.5	45
chopped	1 cup	65	14.8	2.6	.2	17
cooked	1 cup	61	13.7	2.5	.2	15
Onions, green	1 lb	163	37.2	6.8	.9	23
chopped	1 cup	36	8.2	1.5	.2	5
Oranges, raw	1	64	16.0	1.3	.3	1
sections	1 cup	88	22.0	1.8	.4	2
Papaya, raw	1 lb	119	30.4	1.8	.3	9
cubed	1 cup	55	14.0	.8	.1	4
Parsley, raw	1 cup	26	5.1	2.2	.4	27
	1 tbsp	2	.3	.1	tr	2
Parsnips, raw	1 lb	293	67.5	6.6	1.9	46
cooked, diced	1 cup	102	23.1	2.3	.8	12
Peaches, fresh	1 lb	150	38.3	2.4	.4	4
	1 (¼ lb)	33	8.5	.5	.	1
canned	1 cup	76	19.8	1.0	.2	5
Pears, fresh	1 lb.	277	69.4	3.2	1.8	9
D'Anjou	1	122	30.6	1.4	.8	4
canned	1 cup	78	20.3	.5	.5	2
Peas, green, raw	1 lb.	381	65.3	28.6	1.8	9
cooked	1 cup	114	19.4	8.6	.6	2
canned	1 cup	150	28.6	8.0	.7	401
frozen	10-oz pkg	207	36.4	15.3	.9	366
split, dry	1 cup	696	125.4	48.4	2.0	80
Peppers, hot, green, chopped	1 cup	49	12.3	1.7	.2	20
fresh, green, chopped	1 cup	33	7.2	1.8	.3	
canned, pimientos	1 tbsp.	4	.8	.1	.1	

NUTRIENT ANALYSIS OF FRUITS AND VEGETABLES (Cont.)

	Amount	Calories	CHO (gm)	PRO (gm)	Fat (gm)	NA (mg)
Pineapple, raw	1 lb	236	62.1	1.8	.9	5
tidbits, canned	1 cup	96	25.1	.7	.2	2
Plums, damson, raw	1 lb	272	73.5	2.1	tr	8
canned	1 cup	114	29.6	1.0	.5	5
Popcorn, plain, popped	1 cup	23	4.6	.8	.3	tr
Potatoes, raw, pared	1 lb.	259	58.2	7.1	.3	10
raw, diced	1 cup	114	25.7	3.2	.2	5
cooked in skin	1 lb	314	70.6	8.7	.4	12
cooked, diced	1 cup	118	26.5	3.3	.2	5
Prunes, dried, pitted	1 lb	1,157	305.7	9.5	2.7	36
cooked, pitted	1 cup	253	66.7	2.1	.6	9
Pumpkin, canned	16-oz can	150	35.8	4.5	1.4	9
	1 cup	81	19.4	2.5	.7	5
Radishes	1 lb	77	16.3	4.5	.5	82
sliced	1 cup	20	4.1	1.2	.1	21
Raisins	1 cup	419	112.2	3.6	.3	39
	1 tbsp	26	7.0	.2	tr	2
Raspberries, raw, Black	1 cup	98	21.0	2.0	1.9	1
Red	1 cup	70	16.7	1.5	.6	1
Rhubarb, raw	1 lb	62	14.4	2.3	.4	8
diced	1 cup	20	4.5	.7	.1	2
Rutabagas, raw	1 lb	177	42.4	4.2	.4	19
cubed	1 cup	64	15.4	1.5	.1	7
	varies					

Food	Measure					
Salsify, cooked	1 cup	16 to 94	20.4	3.5	.8	
Sauerkraut, canned	1 lb	82	18.1	4.5	.9	3,388
	1 cup	42	9.4	2.4	.5	1,755
Shallots, chopped	1 tbsp	7	1.7	.3	tr	1
Soybeans, raw	1 cup	846	70.4	71.6	37.2	11
cooked	1 cup	234	19.4	19.8	10.3	4
Tofu, curd	1 lb	327	10.9	35.4	19.1	32
Spinach, raw	1 lb.	118	19.5	14.5	1.4	322
chopped	1 cup	14	2.4	1.8	.2	39
cooked	1 cup	41	6.5	5.4	.5	90
canned	1 cup	44	7.0	4.6	.9	548
frozen	10-oz pkg	68	10.8	8.8	.9	162
Squash:						
summer, raw	1 lb	36	19.1	5.0	.5	5
cooked	1 cup	29	6.5	1.9	.2	2
zucchini, raw	1 lb	77	16.3	5.4	.5	5
	1 cup	22	4.7	1.6	.1	1
winter, baked	1 lb	286	69.9	8.2	1.8	5
frozen	1 cup	129	31.6	3.7	.8	2
	12-oz pkg	129	31.3	4.1	1.0	3
Strawberries, raw	1 pint	121	27.4	2.3	1.6	3
	1 lb	168	38.1	3.2	2.3	5
	1 cup	55	12.5	1.0	.7	1
Sunflower seeds, hulled	1 lb	2,540	90.3	108.9	214.6	136

NUTRIENT ANALYSIS OF FRUITS AND VEGETABLES (Cont.)

	Amount	Calories	CHO (gm)	PRO (gm)	Fat (gm)	NA (mg)
Sweet potatoes, raw, pared	1 lb.	517	119.3	7.7	1.8	45
cooked, mashed	1 cup	291	67.1	4.3	1.0	26
baked	1 (5"x2")	161	37.0	2.4	.6	14
yams, raw, with skin	1 lb.	394	90.5	8.2	.8	
Tangerines	1 med	39	10.0	.7	.2	2
Tomatoes, raw, large	1 (3"x2⅛")	40	8.6	2.0	.4	5
medium	(⅓ lb)	27	5.8	1.4	.2	4
canned	1 cup	51	10.4	2.4	.5	313
Tomato						
catsup	1 tbsp	16	3.8	.3	.1	156
paste	6-oz can	139	31.6	5.8	.7	65
1 cup	215	48.7	8.9	1.0	100
purée	29-oz can	321	73.2	14.0	1.6	3,280
1 cup	92	20.9	4.0	.5	937
sauce	1 cup	314	23.8	4.3	23.3	937
Turnips, raw, diced	1 lb	39	8.6	1.3	.3	64
cooked, diced	1 cup	36	7.6	1.2	.3	53
Turnip greens, raw	1 lb.	127	22.7	13.6	1.4	
cooked	1 cup	29	5.2	3.2	.3	
frozen	10-oz pkg	65	11.4	7.4	.9	65
Water chestnuts	1 lb	276	66.4	4.9	.7	70

Watercress, chopped	1 cup	24	3.8	2.8	.4	65
Watermelon	1 lb	118	29.0	2.3	.9	5
	1 cup	42	10.2	.8	.3	2
JUICES						
Apple or cider	1 cup	117	29.5	.2	tr	2
Apricot nectar	1 cup	143	36.6	.8	.3	tr
Grapefruit	1 cup	101	24.2	1.2	.2	2
Grapefruit and orange	1 cup	109	26.0	1.5	.2	tr
Grape	1 cup	167	42.0	.5	tr	5
Lemon	1 tbsp.	4	1.2	.1	tr	tr
Orange	1 cup	122	28.9	1.7	.2	2
Peach nectar	1 cup	120	30.9	.5	tr	2
Pear nectar	1 cup	130	33.0	.8	.5	3
Pineapple	1 cup	138	33.8	1.0	.3	3
Prune	1 cup	197	48.6	1.0	.3	5
Tangelo	1 cup	101	24.0	1.2	.2	
Tangerine	1 cup	106	24.9	1.2	.5	2
Tomato	1 cup	46	10.4	2.2	.2	486

NUTRIENT ANALYSIS OF CONDIMENTS

	Amount	Calories	CHO (gm)	PRO (gm)	Fat (gm)	NA (mg)
Baking powder	1 tsp	4	.9	tr	tr	329
salt-free	1 tsp	7	1.8			tr
Baking soda	1 tsp					1,030
Beef or chicken soup concentrate	1 cube	5	.2	.8	.1	960
	1 tsp	2	.1	.4	.1	480
Catsup	1 tbsp	16	3.8	.3	.1	156
Cocoa	1 cup	224	41.7	14.9	16.3	617
	1 tbsp	14	2.6	.9	1.0	39
Cream of tartar	1 tsp	2	.5	tr	tr	tr
Mustard, prepared						
brown	1 tbsp	15	.9	.9	.9	195
yellow	1 tbsp	12	.9	.6	.6	184
Olives						
green	4 med.	15	tr	tr	2	66
ripe	2 large	15	2	tr	2	73
Salt	1 tsp.					2,132
Soy sauce	1 tbsp	12	1.7	1.0	.2	1,319
Vinegar	1 cup	34	14.2	tr		tr
	1 tbsp	2	.9	tr		tr
Worcestershire sauce	1 tbsp	10	2			200
Yeast						
active dry	1 tbsp	27	3.6	3.5	.1	5
	1 pkg	20	2.7	2.6	.1	4
compressed	1 oz	24	3.1	3.4	.1	5

3
PLANNING FOR
SPECIAL MENUS

Menus can be very helpful when you plan your diabetic diet. Actually, writing it down often helps clarify the relationship of menu items and makes it easier to see the whole thing in perspective.

It is important to eat everything listed in a diabetic daily meal plan. Changes should not be made without first checking with your doctor. You can sometimes save something from a meal for a snack or eat a little earlier or later than scheduled, but even that must be planned in advance.

When I am planning menus I always try to include the following:

Two or three servings of meat, poultry, or fish daily

Three or four servings of fruits and vegetables daily

Three or four servings of whole grain cereals daily

The appropriate amount of milk or other dairy products

Desserts and other less necessary extras are included only after all other needs have been met. Since fiber is helpful to most people, I also try to include as many foods rich in fiber as possible.

All of the necessary ingredients for a well-balanced menu are included in the diabetic daily food plan, so if you are following your food plan you needn't worry about having a balanced diet. I often hear people tell diabetics how well they look, and I think to myself that they would also look that good if they consumed as good a diet as most diabetics do.

When I'm helping diabetics plan their menus, we generally start out with the following guidelines. I always plan menus to fit their tastes and lifestyles; they will be more likely to follow it with no diversions.

BASIC DAILY FOOD EXCHANGE ALLOWANCE AT DIFFERENT CALORIC LEVELS

Exchanges	1200	1400	1600	1800	2000
Breakfast					
Bread or starch	2	2	2	2	2
Fruit	1	1	2	2	2
Skim milk	1	1	1	1	1
Fat	1	1	1	1	1
Lunch or dinner at noon					
Bread or starch	2	2	2	2	3
Fruit	1	1	1	1	1
Skim milk	0	0	0	½	½
Lean meat	3	3	3	3	3
Vegetable	1	1	1	1	1
Fat	1	1	1	2	2
Dinner or supper in the evening					
Bread or starch	1	2	2	3	3
Fruit	1	1	1	1	1
Skim milk	0	0	0	½	½
Lean meat	2	2	3	3	3
Vegetable	1	2	2	2	2
Fat	0	1	1	1	1
Evening snack					
Bread or starch	0	0	1	1	1
Fruit	1	1	1	1	2
Skim milk	1	1	1	1	1
Fat	0	0	0	0	1

This menu plan is based on bread/starch exchanges. However, just because the menu plan lists 5 bread exchanges doesn't mean that you should include five slices of bread in your menu. Those bread exchanges should also be used for other things such as baked potatoes, starchy vegetables, and high-fiber bran muffins; of course, you can use part of them for some simple desserts such as ice milk, frozen yogurt, and angel food cake.

The number of exchanges for each diet is based on the following table, which lists the number of exchanges for different caloric levels and the percentages of carbohydrate (CHO), protein (PRO), and fat (FAT) included at the different levels. As you see, the table follows the high-carbohydrate, low-fat, and moderate-protein diet recommended by The American Diabetic Association, Inc., and the American Dietetic Association.

After the basic menu is planned, it must be extended to provide a diet modification at each level of the diabetic diet. I have extended the following menus as I would have extended them at work, with a column for each of the levels of the diet. To read the menu, find the diet heading that you need and then plan to use everything in that column for your diet for that meal. Some foods are free and you can use as much of them as you like—that is indicated, as well as the portion size for each item.

I hope you will find the following menus useful and that they will help you find ways to include new items—especially the recipes in this book—in your own diet plans.

MENU PLAN FOR DIABETIC DIETS

Exchanges	1200	1400	1600	1800	2000
Starch/bread	5	6	7	8	9
Lean meat	5	5	6	6	6
Vegetable	2	3	3	3	3
Fruit	4	4	5	5	6
Skim milk	2	2	2	3	3
Fat	2	3	3	4	5
Total calories	1235	1385	1580	1795	1980
Percentages					
CHO	57	57	55	58	58
PRO	24	23	23	22	21
FAT	19	20	22	20	21
Total percent	100	100	100	100	100

NEW YEAR'S DAY—Dinner at noon

Fruit Soup* with Melba toast rounds
Baked ham
Escalloped potatoes
Creole Green Beans*
Tossed vegetable salad with Vinaigrette Dressing*
Stewed Cranberries*
Relish tray (dill pickles, celery, and carrot sticks)
Skim milk, coffee, or tea
Lemon Pie*

Food Item	1200	1400	1600	1800	2000
Fruit Soup	½ cup at all levels of the diet				
Melba toast rounds					5
Baked ham	3 ounces at all levels of the diet				
Escalloped potatoes	½ cup at all levels of the diet				
Creole Green Beans	½ cup at all levels of the diet				
Tossed vegetable salad	as desired at all levels of the diet				
Vinaigrette Dressing	2 tablespoons at all levels of the diet				
Stewed Cranberries	½ cup at all levels of the diet				
Relish tray	as desired at all levels of the diet				
Skim milk				4 oz	4 oz
Margarine				1 tsp	1 tsp
Lemon Pie	⅛ pie at all levels of the diet				
Coffee or tea	as desired at all levels of the diet				

Menu notes: Beans were included because it is considered lucky to eat them on New Year's Day in some parts of the country.

*See Index.

LABOR DAY PICNIC—at noon

**Hamburger on a bun with lettuce, catsup, mustard, and
  pickle relish**
Potato Salad*
Pickled Vegetables*
Tossed salad with Vinaigrette Dressing*
Cubed fresh watermelon
Skim milk, coffee, tea, or Sparkling Punch*
Buttermilk Cookies*

Food Item	1200	1400	1600	1800	2000
Hamburger, raw weight	4 ounces at all levels of the diet				
Hamburger bun	1 small at all levels of the diet				
Margarine				1 tsp	1 tsp
Lettuce	as desired at all levels of the diet				
Catsup	1 tablespoon at all levels of the diet				
Mustard	1 teaspoon at all levels of the diet				
Pickle relish	1 teaspoon at all levels of the diet				
Potato Salad	½ cup at all levels of the diet				
Pickled Vegetables	½ cup at all levels of the diet				
Tossed vegetable salad	as desired at all levels of the diet				
Vinaigrette Dressing	2 tablespoons at all levels of the diet				
Cubed watermelon	1 cup at all levels of the diet				
Skim milk				4 oz	4 oz
Buttermilk cookies					2
Coffee, tea, or Sparkling Punch	as desired at all levels of the diet				

Menu notes: The tossed salad should be something beautiful, with fresh vegetables that are low in carbohydrate so everyone can eat all they want of it. It might include broccoli spears, cauliflower slices, mushrooms, green peppers julienne, a little red cabbage—anything that is colorful, fresh, and low in calories—along with fresh crisp lettuce or other greens such as escarole or spinach.

*See Index.

THANKSGIVING—Dinner at noon

Tomato Bouillon*
Roast Turkey*
Bread Dressing*
Turkey Gravy*
Baked sweet potato
Broccoli
Cranberry Gelatin* with Kay's Cooked Dressing*
Relish plate (green pepper strips, dill pickles, carrot and
    celery strips)
Skim milk, coffee, or tea
Pumpkin Scotch Pie* with Whipped Topping*

Food Item	1200	1400	1600	1800	2000
Tomato Bouillon	1 cup at all levels of the diet					
Roast Turkey	3 ounces cooked weight at all levels of the diet				
Bread Dressing					1 square
Turkey Gravy	¼ cup at all levels of the diet				
Baked sweet potato	1 small at all levels of the diet				
Broccoli	½ cup at all levels of the diet				
Cranberry Gelatin	1 square at all levels of the diet				
Kay's Cooked Dressing	1 tablespoon at all levels of the diet				
Relish plate	as desired at all levels of the diet				
Margarine				1 tsp	
Skim milk				4 oz	4 oz
Pumpkin Scotch Pie	⅛ pie at all levels of the diet				
Whipped Topping	2 tablespoons at all levels of the diet				
Coffee or tea	as desired at all levels of the diet				
Fruit exchange for afternoon snack	1 at all levels of the diet				

*See Index.

CHRISTMAS DAY—Dinner at noon

Hot Beef Bouillon*
Roast Beef*
Mashed potatoes
Brown Gravy*
Stewed Cranberries*
Cauliflower
Relish plate (Mrs. Riley's Pickles*, carrot and celery sticks)
Banana gelatin with Kay's Cooked Dressing*
Small plain roll
Margarine
Skim milk, coffee, or tea
Strawberry Chiffon Pie*

Food Item	1200	1400	1600	1800	2000
Hot Beef Bouillon	1 cup at all levels of the diet				
Roast Beef	3 ounces at all levels of the diet				
Mashed potatoes	½ cup at all levels of the diet				
Brown Gravy	¼ cup at all levels of the diet				
Stewed Cranberries	½ cup at all levels of the diet				
Cauliflower	½ cup at all levels of the diet				
Relish plate	as desired at all levels of the diet				
Banana gelatin	1 serving at all levels of the diet				
Kay's Cooked Dressing	1 tablespoon at all levels of the diet				
Small plain roll					1
Margarine				1 tsp	1 tsp
Skim milk				4 oz	4 oz
Strawberry Chiffon Pie	⅛ pie at all levels of the diet				
Coffee or tea	as desired at all levels of the diet				

Menu notes: Prepare banana gelatin by using ½ banana per person in Fruit-Flavored Gelatin.*

Use recipe for beef broth to prepare Beef Bouillon.

See Index.

BREAKFAST

Orange or grapefruit juice
Cereal
Skim milk
Bran Muffin*
Coffee or tea

Food Item	1200	1400	1600	1800	2000
Orange or grapefruit juice	4 ounces at all levels of the diet				
½ cup cooked or ¾ cup unsweetened prepared cereal	1 serving at all levels of the diet				
Skim milk	8 ounces at all levels of the diet				
Bran Muffin	1 at all levels of the diet				
Coffee or tea	as desired at all levels of the diet				
Fruit exchange for morning snack			1	1	1

Menu notes: The Bran Muffin may also be saved for a morning snack, if desired. If you choose a bran muffin that includes only ½ fat exchange, the remaining ½ fat exchange could be margarine or ½ serving of Cinnamon Spread.*

*See Index.

BREAKFAST

Orange juice
Sliced fresh peaches
Shredded wheat
Cinnamon Roll*
Margarine
Skim milk
Coffee or tea

Food Item	1200	1400	1600	1800	2000
Orange juice			4 oz	4 oz	4 oz
Sliced unsweetened fresh, frozen, or canned peaches	½ cup at all levels of the diet				
Shredded wheat	1 large biscuit at all levels of the diet				
Cinnamon Roll	1 at all levels of the diet				
Margarine	½ teaspoon at all levels of the diet				
Skim milk	8 ounces at all levels of the diet				
Coffee or tea	as desired at all levels of the diet				

Menu notes: 1 slice whole wheat toast and 1 teaspoon margarine may be substituted for the Cinnamon Roll and ½ teaspoon margarine.

*See Index.

BREAKFAST

Applesauce
Orange juice
Oat Bran Pancakes*
Cinnamon Shake*
Skim milk
Coffee or milk

Food Item	1200	1400	1600	1800	2000
Unsweetened applesauce	½ cup at all levels of the diet				
Orange juice			4 oz	4 oz	4 oz
Oat Bran Pancakes	2 at all levels of the diet				
Cinnamon Shake	as desired at all levels of the diet				
Skim milk	8 ounces at all levels of the diet				
Coffee or tea	as desired at all levels of the diet				

Menu notes: The applesauce may be warmed and served over the pancakes or ¼ cup low-calorie pancake syrup may also be used.

See Index.

VEGETABLE BEEF SOUP—evening

Vegetable Beef Soup* with Melba toast rounds
Lettuce salad with Spicy Tomato Dressing*
Mrs. Riley's Pickles*
Plain roll
Vanilla ice milk
Chocolate Sauce*
Unsweetened pineapple
Skim milk
Coffee or tea

Food Item	1200	1400	1600	1800	2000
Vegetable Beef Soup	¾ cup	¾ cup	1 cup	1 cup	1 cup
Melba toast rounds	5	8	8	8	8
Lettuce salad	as desired at all levels of the diet				
Spicy Tomato Dressing	2 tablespoons at all levels of the diet				
Mrs. Riley's Pickles	up to ¼ cup at all levels of the diet				
Small plain roll				1	1
Vanilla ice milk		½ cup	½ cup	½ cup	½ cup
Chocolate Sauce		2 tbsp	2 tbsp	2 tbsp	2 tbsp
Unsweetened pineapple	½ cup at all levels of the diet				
Skim milk				4 oz	4 oz
Coffee or tea	as desired at all levels of the diet				

*See Index.

SOUP AND SANDWICH—at noon

Tomato Bouillon* with Melba toast rounds
Chicken Sandwich Spread* on Rich Whole Wheat Bread*
Relish plate (sliced dill pickles, green pepper sticks, radishes)
Three-Bean Salad*
Fresh pear
Skim milk, coffee, or tea

Food Item	1200	1400	1600	1800	2000
Tomato Bouillon	1 cup at all levels of the diet				
Melba toast rounds					5
Chicken Sandwich Spread	⅓ cup at all levels of the diet				
Rich Whole Wheat Bread	2 slices at all levels of the diet				
Miracle Whip salad dressing	2 tsp	2 tsp	2 tsp	4 tsp	4 tsp
Lettuce for sandwich	as desired at all levels of the diet				
Relish plate	as desired at all levels of the diet				
Three-Bean Salad	½ cup at all levels of the diet				
Pear	1 small fresh or canned at all levels of the diet				
Skim milk				4 oz	4 oz
Coffee or tea	as desired at all levels of the diet				

Menu notes: Three ounces of sliced turkey or chicken with fat and gristle removed may be substituted for the Chicken Sandwich Spread, if desired. Two teaspoons of Miracle Whip salad dressing is equal to 1 teaspoon margarine; margarine may be substituted, if desired.

*See Index.

SALAD LUNCHEON—at noon

Hot Beef Bouillon* with Melba toast rounds
Chef's Salad*
Raisin Bread*
Cinnamon Spread*
Cole Slaw*
Skim milk
Pineapple Gelatin*
Whipped Topping*
Coffee or tea

Food Item	1200	1400	1600	1800	2000
Hot Beef Bouillon	as desired ounces at all levels of the diet				
Melba toast rounds					5
Chef's Salad with 1 extra ounce meat or chicken	1 serving at all levels of the diet				
Raisin Bread	1 slice at all levels of the diet				
Cinnamon Spread or	1½ tbsp	1½ tbsp	1½ tbsp	1 tbsp	1 tbsp
Margarine	1 tsp	1 tsp	1 tsp	2 tsp	2 tsp
Cole Slaw	½ cup at all levels of the diet				
Skim milk				4 oz	4 oz
Pineapple Gelatin	1 serving at all levels of the diet				
Whipped Topping	2 tablespoons at all levels of the diet				
Coffee or tea	as desired at all levels of the diet				

Menu notes: Prepare Pineapple Gelatin using ½ cup crushed, canned unsweetened pineapple per serving. As much gelatin as desired may be used per serving.

Use recipe for Beef Broth to prepare Beef Bouillon.

Raisin Bread may be toasted or served at room temperature.

*See Index.

FISH FOR DINNER OR SUPPER—evening

Baked Halibut Steak* with Tartar Sauce*
Broccoli Rice Casserole*
Steamed carrots
Baked potato
Plain roll
Unsweetened fresh or frozen strawberries
Skim milk, coffee, or tea

Food Item	1200	1400	1600	1800	2000
Baked Halibut Steak, cooked weight	2 oz	2 oz	3 oz	3 oz	3 oz
Tartar Sauce	up to 2 tablespoons at all levels of the diet				
Broccoli Rice Casserole			½ cup	½ cup	½ cup	½ cup
Steamed carrots	½ cup				
Baked potato	1 small	1 medium	1 medium	1 medium	1 medium
Small plain roll				1	1
Unsweetened fresh or frozen strawberries	1¼ cups at all levels of the diet				
Skim milk				4 oz	4 oz
Coffee or tea	as desired at all levels of the diet				

Menu notes: Strawberries may be molded in unsweetened fruit gelatin, if desired, at all levels of the diet.

*See Index.

MINESTRONE SOUP—evening

Minestrone Soup* with Melba toast rounds
Cole Slaw*
Blueberries or blackberries
Plain roll
Key Lime Pie*
Skim milk, coffee, or tea

Food Item	1200	1400	1600	1800	2000
Minestrone Soup	1 cup at all levels of the diet				
Melba toast rounds	2	5	5	5	5
Extra ounce(s) of lean meat to be added to each serving of soup	1 oz	1 oz	2 oz	2 oz	2 oz
Cole Slaw	½ cup at all levels of the diet				
Unsweetened fresh or frozen blueberries or blackberries	¾ cup at all levels of the diet				
Small plain roll				1	1
Key Lime Pie		⅛ pie	⅛ pie	⅛ pie	⅛ pie
Skim milk				4 oz	4 oz
Coffee or tea	as desired at all levels of the diet				

*See Index.

SOUP AND SANDWICH—evening

Swiss* or Mulligatawny* Soup
Roast beef sandwich on Three-Grain Bread*
Frijole Salad*
Cantaloupe cubes
Skim milk, coffee, or tea

Food Item	1200	1400	1600	1800	2000
Swiss Soup	1 cup	1 cup			
Mulligatawny Soup			1 cup	1 cup	1 cup
Roast beef	2 ounces at all levels of the diet				
Three-Grain Bread	1 slice	2 slices	1 slice	2 slices	2 slices
Miracle Whip salad dressing		2 tsp	2 tsp	2 tsp	2 tsp
or margarine		1 tsp	1 tsp	1 tsp	1 tsp
Mustard	as desired at all levels of the diet				
Frijole salad	½ cup	1 cup	1 cup	1 cup	1 cup
Cantaloupe cubes	1 cup at all levels of the diet				
Skim milk				4 oz	4 oz
Coffee or tea	as desired at all levels of the diet				

Menu notes: The 1200-calorie level of the diet cannot have the Miracle Whip or margarine so you might want to try Creamy Garlic Dressing* or Yogurt Topping* in your sandwich.

*See Index.

BREAKFAST

Orange juice
Cereal
Skim milk
Coffee or tea

MORNING COFFEE WITH FRIENDS

Chocolate Nut Bread*
Pastel Cookie*
Fresh fruit cup with Orange Liqueur*
Coffee or tea

Food Item	1200	1400	1600	1800	2000
Breakfast					
Orange juice			4 oz	4 oz	4 oz
½ cup cooked or ¾ cup unsweetened prepared cereal	1 serving at all levels of the diet				
Skim milk	8 oz at all levels of the diet				
Coffee or tea	as desired at all levels of the diet				
Morning Coffee with Friends					
Chocolate Nut Bread	½ slice at all levels of the diet				
Pastel Cookie	1 at all levels of the diet				
Fresh fruit cup	½ cup fruit with ½ teaspoon Orange Liqueur at all levels of the diet				
Coffee or tea	as desired at all levels of the diet				

Menu notes: The Chocolate Nut Bread and 1 Pastel Cookie give you 1 bread and 1 fat exchange. You can substitute any other foods that total 1 bread and 1 fat exchange for your morning coffee, if desired.

I have included this and the next menu to show that you can save food from a meal to use as a snack in the morning, afternoon, or evening. However, this is meant to be a guide and should be changed according to your own schedule. Non-insulin-dependent persons have more leeway in their diet than do insulin-dependent persons. If you are insulin dependent, you should check with your doctor or dietitian before attempting any drastic reduction in any of your menus.

See Index.

LUNCH OR DINNER—at noon

Broiled round steak
Stir-Fry Tomatoes*
Lettuce salad with Creamy Garlic Dressing*
Applesauce
Skim milk, coffee, or tea

AFTERNOON TEA

Devil's Food Cake* with Fluffy Frosting*
High-Fiber Cookies*
Graham crackers
Sparkling Punch*
Coffee or tea

Food Item	1200	1400	1600	1800	2000
Lunch or Dinner at Noon					
Broiled round steak		3 ounces cooked weight at all levels of the diet			
Stir-Fry Tomatoes		about ¾ cup at all levels of the diet			
Lettuce salad		as desired at all levels of the diet			
Creamy Garlic Dressing		up to 2 tablespoons at all levels of the diet			
Unsweetened applesauce		½ cup at all levels of the diet			
Skim milk				4 oz	4 oz
Coffee or tea		as desired at all levels of the diet			
Afternoon Tea					
Devil's Food Cake		1 square at all levels of the diet			
Fluffy Frosting		1½ tablespoons at all levels of the diet			
High-Fiber Cookies				1	1
Graham crackers	3	3	3		3
Sparkling Punch		as desired at all levels of the diet			
Coffee or tea		as desired at all levels of the diet			

See Index.

Menu notes: This menu does not have to be followed exactly but can serve as a guide. You can substitute other foods with the same exchange values for any food in the menu or you can add free foods such as relish plate of free food in the afternoon as long as you stay within the guidelines for your diet.

It is easier to control the menu when you serve it in your own home, but you can remember food exchanges and maintain your own diet if you are careful when you go to parties.

If finger sandwiches are served, pick ones with a plain filling and consider each finger sandwich as ½ bread exchange if it is a double sandwich with the crusts trimmed off and with a plain filling.

4
CHOLESTEROL

Recent research indicates that about 75 percent of all diabetics die of atherosclerosis or related diseases. Since the American Medical Association, The American Diabetes Association, Inc., The American Diatetic Association, and the American Heart Association all stress that a low-cholesterol count below 200 will lessen the danger of atherosclerosis, it is only logical that diabetics should reevaluate their diets in light of these findings.

I think that anyone following a low-cholesterol diet should emphasize a high-fiber diet with particular attention to water-soluble fiber, such as that found in oat bran, seeds, and fruits. I have known several people who have lowered their cholesterol counts dramatically when they added oat bran to their diets, so I recommend a substantial intake of oat bran for anyone trying to control his or her cholesterol count. I have included several recipes using oat bran, which I hope you will use in your diet. I also recommend using it as a cereal. When making hot oatmeal cereal, I like to combine one-half oat bran and one-half oatmeal prepared according to the directions for preparing oatmeal.

The low-cholesterol diet isn't hard to follow, and it is simple to plan your diabetic diet using the low-cholesterol guidelines. They both emphasize decreased sugar and fat with a moderate amount of meat and increased complex carbohydrates.

We have been using a low-cholesterol diet at our house for years since our doctor put my husband, Chuck, on a low-cholesterol diet when he was forty-three. Since I have always cooked all of our food following low-cholesterol guidelines, I didn't have to make any changes in my diet when I discovered I should be on a low-cholesterol diet because of my diabetes.

Since it is very important that you follow a low-cholesterol diet if you are diabetic, I am including the following information from the American Heart Association from their brochure "The American Heart Association Diet: An Eating Plan for Healthy Americans."

THE GOALS OF THE AHA DIET

This plan outlines a wholesome eating style for a healthy, active life while reducing the amount of cholesterol in your blood to the level safest for your heart. The AHA diet can help you:

- Meet your daily requirements for protein, vitamins, minerals, and other nutrients
- Achieve and maintain your desirable weight
- Reduce your total intake of fat to about 30 percent of calories
- Avoid eating too many foods containing saturated fat and cholesterol
- Substitute polyunsaturated fat for saturated fat whenever possible and yet not eat too much of any kind of fat

Make these changes gradually over a period of several months so they become a natural part of your permanent eating pattern.

The American Heart Association recommends this diet for all Americans over the age of two. Ask your doctor for specific advice before making major eating pattern changes in young children. Consult your doctor or nutritionist about the nutrient needs of children and teenagers during growth periods, and get advice about the special nutritional needs of women who are pregnant or breast feeding.

GUIDELINES

The American Heart Association has developed the following guidelines for the low-cholesterol diet, all of which will fit very easily into your present diabetic diet plan.

Atherosclerosis

Atherosclerosis is a slowly developing process in which the lining of the arteries becomes coated with fatty substances such as cholesterol (lipid deposits). These deposits result in narrowing and scarring of the channels through which the blood flows. Eventually an artery may close off completely, either because the deposits have grown together or because a blood clot plugs up the narrowed passage. Whenever an artery is blocked, damage occurs in the part of the body that the blocked artery supplies. If the blockage occurs in an artery serving the heart muscle (a coronary artery), a heart attack can result. If it occurs in an artery supplying the brain, a stroke can occur. We have good evidence that most people, including those who have a family history of heart or high blood cholesterol, can reduce the risk of having a heart attack by following a cholesterol-lowering plan. You can also cut your heart attack risk by not smoking and by getting medical treatment to control high blood pressure or diabetes.

Cholesterol

Too much cholesterol in the circulatory system encourages the development of heart and blood vessel diseases.

We get cholesterol in two ways: it is manufactured by the body from all foods, and we get it directly from foods of animal origin.

Egg yolks and organ meats are very high in cholesterol, and shrimp, lobster, and sardines are moderately high in the substance. There is no cholesterol in foods of plant origin such as fruits, vegetables, grains, cereals, seeds, and nuts, and these foods are highly recommended.

Saturated Fats

Saturated fats tend to raise the level of cholesterol in the blood. These are fats that harden at room temperature, and they are found in most animal products and some hydrogenated vegetable products.

Saturated animal fats are found in beef, lamb, pork, and ham; in shortenings, and in coconut oil, cocoa butter, and palm oil (used in commercially prepared cookies, pie fillings, and nondairy milk and cream substitutes). They are sometimes advertised as cholesterol-free, which is true. *However*, they are very high in saturated fat and should be avoided. These oils are often used in store-brought bakery products, candies, fried foods, and milk and cream substitutes. Read labels carefully to avoid these products.

Low-Fat Meats

Total fat is low in chicken, turkey, fish, and lean veal, and they are recommended.

Polyunsaturated Fats

Polyunsaturated fats are usually liquid oils of vegetable origin. Oils such as corn, cottonseed, safflower, sesame seed, soybean, and sunflower seed are high in polyunsaturated fat. These oils help lower the level of blood cholesterol by aiding the body in getting rid of excessive newly formed cholesterol.

Olive oil and peanut oil are also vegetable products, but they are low in polyunsaturated fats. Your daily use of salad dressings, cooking fats, and margarines should emphasize the polyunsaturated vegetable oils.

Hydrogenation

Hydrogenation changes liquid fats to solid fats. Completely hydrogenated (hardened) oils resemble saturated fats and should be avoided or used in moderation; but most margarines and shortenings containing partially hydrogenated oils are acceptable if their labels say they contain twice as much polyunsaturated as saturated fat.

To Control Your Intake of Cholesterol-Rich Foods

- Eat no more than two egg yolks a week, *including* eggs used in cooking.
- Limit your use of organ meats, shrimp, lobster, and sardines.

To Control the Amount and Type of What You Eat

- Use fish, chicken or turkey without the skin, and veal in most of your meat exchanges for the week. Use moderate-size portions of beef, lamb, pork, and ham less frequently. Limit your intake of meat, seafood, and poultry to no more than 5–7 ounces per day.
- Choose lean cuts of meat, trim visible fat, and discard fat that cooks out of the meat. Substitute meatless or low-meat main dishes for regular entrees.
- Avoid deep-fat frying; use cooking methods that help to remove fat— baking, broiling, boiling, roasting, and stewing.
- Restrict your use of "luncheon" and "variety" meats like sausages and salami.

- Instead of butter and other cooking fats that are solid or completely hydrogenated, use liquid vegetable oils and margarines that are rich in polyunsaturated fats. Use no more than 5–8 teaspoons of fats and oils per day, including those used in cooking, baking, and salads.
- Instead of whole milk and cheeses made from whole milk and cream, use skim milk and skim milk cheeses.

Limit Your Salt Intake

- Most Americans use 10–15 times more salt than they need.

THE AHA DIET

Vegetables and Fruits

Vegetables and fruits are high in vitamins, minerals, potassium, and fiber. They contain no cholesterol and are low in fat, calories, and sodium. Almost all vegetables and fruits are "OKAY foods" and should be part of your daily food plan. You should include at least one serving from the high-vitamin-C list daily and at least one serving from the high-vitamin-A list several times weekly; include other fruits and vegetables according to your diet plan.

When you are reducing your intake of red meat and egg yolks, you can increase your iron intake by eating more leafy green vegetables, peas and beans (fresh and dried), dried fruits, and whole-grain and enriched cereals. Your body can make better use of the iron these foods provide if you eat a good source of vitamin C with them.

High vitamin C vegetables and fruits:

- Asparagus
- Broccoli
- Cabbage
- Cantaloupe
- Grapefruit
- Greens
- Green pepper
- Oranges
- Potatoes
- Spinach
- Strawberries
- Tangerines
- Tomatoes

High vitamin A fruits and vegetables:

- Broccoli
- Cantaloupe
- Carrots
- Greens
- Peaches
- Pumpkin
- Spinach
- Sweet potatoes
- Winter squash

Fruits and vegetables to avoid:

- Coconut

Milk Products

Milk products are high in protein, phosphorus, niacin, riboflavin, and vitamins A and D. Most diabetic diets include skim milk and low-fat dry milk or buttermilk.

OKAY milk products:

- Yogurt made from skim milk
- Buttermilk made from skim milk
- Drinks made with skim or low-fat milk
- Ice milk
- Sherbet
- Frozen low-fat yogurt
- Look for products labeled "fortified with vitamins A and D"

Milk products to avoid:

- Whole milk
- 2% milk
- Dried whole milk
- Buttermilk or yogurt made from whole milk
- Condensed milk
- Evaporated whole milk
- Ice cream
- Cream of all kinds

- Nondairy cream substitutes, unless labeled "made from polyunsaturated fat"
- All cheeses with more than 2 grams of fat per ounce, such as cream cheese, creamed cottage cheese, and most other natural and processed cheeses, such as American, Swiss, mozzarella, and bleu.

Breads, Cereals, Pasta, and Starchy Vegetables

Breads, cereals, pasta, and starchy vegetables are low in fat and cholesterol and high in B vitamins, iron, and fiber. In moderate portions, they are not extremely high in calories; it's the fat and sauces added to them that run up the total calories.

Stretch your meat allowance and your budget by combining small portions of poultry, fish, or meat with vegetables, herbs, and rice or pasta.

OKAY foods in this group:

- Low-fat breads such as wheat, rye, raisin, and white. Those with enriched flours are best.
- Low-fat rolls such as English muffins, frankfurter and hamburger rolls, bagels (except egg bagels), pita bread, and tortillas that are not fried.
- Low-fat crackers and snacks such as animal, graham, rye, saltines, oyster, and matzo crackers; store-bought fig bars; ginger snap and molasses cookies; bread sticks; melba toast; rusks and flatbread; pretzels and popcorn made with approved fat.
- Hot or cold cereals, all kinds except granola-type cereals with coconut, coconut oil, or palm oil.
- Rice and pasta of all kinds except those made with egg yolks.
- Starchy vegetables such as potatoes, lima beans, green peas, winter squash, corn, yams, or sweet potatoes.
- Quick breads such as those made at home with approved fats, oils, and milk products. Use your weekly allowance of 2 egg yolks or try 2 egg whites in place of a whole egg in your favorite recipes.
- Low-fat soups such as broth, bouillon, chicken noodle, tomato-based seafood, minestrone, onion, split pea, tomato, and vegetarian vegetable. Use the canned or powdered varieties, but read labels to choose the ones lowest in fat. Better yet, make soups at home so that you can avoid salt, fat, cream, whole milk, and cheese.

Foods to avoid:

- Products made with egg yolks or with nonapproved fats or oils and whole-milk products
- Butter rolls, egg breads, egg bagels, cheese breads, croissants, commercial doughnuts, muffins, sweet rolls, biscuits, waffles, pancakes, buttered popcorn, and store-bought mixes.
- High-fat commercial crackers such as cheese crackers, butter crackers, and those made with coconut or palm oil.
- Pasta, rice, and vegetables prepared with whole eggs, cream sauce, or high-fat cheese or fried in nonapproved fats.
- Cream soups, vichysoisse, and chunky-style soups that have large amounts of meat in them.

Meat, Poultry, Seafood, Nuts, Dried Beans and Peas, and Eggs

These foods provide protein, B vitamins, iron, and other minerals. *OKAY foods in this group:*

- Chicken and turkey with the fat and skin removed.
- Lean beef, veal, pork, and lamb trimmed of all visible fat.
- Fish and shellfish, all kinds but limit the use of shrimp, lobster, or sardines to no more than one serving of these per week.
- Meatless or low-meat main dishes. Try recipes with dried beans, peas, lentils, tofu (soybean curd), peanut butter, or low-fat cheese instead of meat a few times a week. Also try combining small amounts of meat, fish, or poultry with rice or pasta in mixed dishes or casseroles.
- Egg whites but limit whole eggs or egg yolks to 2 per week.
- Wild game: rabbit, pheasant, venison, wild duck, and other wild game animals generally have less fat than animals raised for the market.
- Instead of high-fat luncheon meats, choose low-fat processed meats with labels showing no more than 2 grams of fat per ounce such as turkey or chicken roll, turkey pastrami, or leaned broiled ham.
- Buy only leanest ground beef, labeled as containing no more than 15 percent fat. Ask your butcher for the fat content if it isn't noted on the label.
- Skim the fat off meat juices before adding to stews, soups, and gravies. Chilling the meat first makes it easier to remove the fat.

Foods to avoid:

- Prime grades of meat and other heavily marbled fatty meats such as corned beef, regular pastrami, short ribs, spare ribs, rib-eye roast or steak, regular ground meat, frankfurters, sausage, bacon, and high-fat luncheon meats
- Goose and domestic duck
- All organ meats and chitterlings; however, liver is so rich in iron and vitamins that a small serving of about 3 ounces is recommended about once a month.

Fats and Oils

Fats and oils are high in vitamins A or E, but all are high in fats and calories. Remember to count the hidden fats in bakery products and snack foods, in cooking, and on vegetables and breads. Use cooking styles that use little or no fat. Try roasting, boiling, or steaming instead of frying.

OKAY fats and oils:

- Vegetable oils listed here by highest to lowest polyunsaturated fat content: safflower, sunflower, corn, and partially hydrogenated soybean and cottonseed oils.
- Margarines: stick, tube, squeeze. One of the OKAY vegetable oils should be listed as the first ingredient on the label with twice as much polyunsaturated fat as saturated fat.
- Salad dressings and mayonnaise (homemade or store-bought) made with OKAY oil; low-calorie dressings can be used as desired.
- Seeds and nuts: all seeds (pumpkin, sesame, sunflower) and most nuts except cashew, macadamia, and pistachio.
- Avocados and olives. Use only in small amounts.
- Peanut butter.

Foods to avoid:

- Solid fat and shortenings, butter, bacon drippings, ham hocks, lard, salt pork, meat fat and drippings, gravy from meat drippings, shortening, suet, and margarines except those listed as OKAY.
- Chocolate, coconut, coconut oil, palm oil, or palm kernel oil. These are often used in bakery products, nondairy creamers, whipped toppings, candy, and commercially fried foods. Read labels carefully.
- Olive and peanut oils.

Desserts, Beverages, and Snacks

These items can be consumed only within the framework of the diabetic diet. They should be chosen from foods that are OKAY for a low-cholesterol diet if you can afford the exchanges.

- First choice items that are low in calories include raw vegetables, fresh fruit, fruit canned or frozen without sugar, sugar-free gelatin, tea, coffee, and cocoa powder.
- Second choice foods that are low in saturated fat and fairly low in calories include dried fruits, seeds, OKAY nuts, plain popcorn, OKAY pretzels, crackers or cookies, sherbet, ice milk, frozen or fruited low-fat yogurt, and angel food cake.
- Other choices include diabetic desserts made with little or no sugar and low-fat milk products.
- Alcoholic beverages should be consumed in moderation and within the framework of your diabetic diet.

Foods to avoid:

- All those not acceptable on your diabetic diet as well as store-bought cakes, pies, cookies, and mixes.
- Coconut.
- High-fat snacks such as deep fried chips and rich crackers.
- Desserts or snacks containing cheese.
- Cream or whole milk.
- Ice cream.

Please note that the above information, which has been taken from a brochure published by the American Heart Association, has been slightly modified to leave out foods that are not acceptable on a diabetic diet. However, the spirit of the diet has been followed exactly, and I have not added any foods that are not approved for a low-cholesterol diet by the American Heart Association.

5
FIBER IN THE DIABETIC DIET

It has been common knowledge for years that a high-fiber diet with plenty of liquid will help prevent constipation, but it is only recently that research has indicated a high-fiber diet that includes a substantial proportion of water-soluble fiber will also help control blood sugar and cholesterol.

Dietary fiber is a general term for the indigestible carbohydrates, including pectin, cellulose, hemicellulose, and lignin, which make up the cell walls of plants. Many foods contain fiber, but it is found most abundantly in raw leafy, root, and tough-skinned vegetables; edible seeds; nuts; fruits; and the outer layer of grains. Because our digestive system does not contain the essential bacteria that breaks down this fiber, it remains more or less unchanged and is passed out of the body through the gastrointestinal system. Dietary fibers have a large capacity to hold water, which gives bulk and softness to the stool and enables food to pass more quickly through the digestive system.

There are two main forms of fiber, water-soluble and water-insoluble. Water-soluble fiber forms a gel in water and is found in oats, beans, seeds, and fruits, especially apples and citrus fruits. Water-soluble dietary fiber helps control cholesterol and blood sugar. Water-insoluble dietary fiber is the kind we generally associate with the word *fiber* and is found in wheat bran, corn bran, whole grains, and vegetables. It, along with liquid, forms bulky stools that travel faster through the intestines and help prevent constipation.

Most nutritionists agree that 30 to 40 grams of dietary fiber per day will give you the best results; the average person gets only about 20 grams of dietary fiber per day. Most diabetics are on a moderately high-fiber diet already since we routinely eat a lot of fruits and vegetables. If you eat whole-grain bread, four or five servings of fruit, and two or three servings of vegetables per day, you are probably already consuming a good amount of fiber. However, in view of the positive results that have been achieved through the consumption of oat bran, it is probably advisable for you to add oat bran to your diet. Check with your doctor first; with his or her approval, use oat bran two or three times daily as a cereal, in muffins or other breads, or added to other recipes. And don't forget to drink at least six to eight glasses of water daily.

Fiber is not easily destroyed. A little water-soluble fiber may be lost in cooking, but it is not destroyed by canning for freezing. However, a lot of fiber is lost when fruits and vegetables are peeled, so don't discard the peelings from apples and do eat the skin from your potato. Your mother was right when she told you they were good for you. Dietary fiber is also specially good for diabetics because foods high in fiber, except for dried beans, are generally more filling than other foods and tend to give you a full feeling after eating them.

I emphasize the importance of oat bran in a diabetic and low-cholesterol diet. One reason we are revising this book is not only because we needed to use the 1986 food exchange lists but also because I wanted to include some oat bran recipes and tell you how important the use of a substantial amount of oat bran can be for the diabetic diet. I have been preaching the ability of oat bran to control blood sugar and cholesterol to the point that I think my friends are getting tired of the subject. I have been successful in getting a lot of people to incorporate oat bran into their daily diet. In this revision I have included several new recipes that use oat bran. I hope you will try them.

Please be cautious in the addition of dietary fiber to your diet if you aren't using much of it now. Although it helps to lower blood sugar and cholesterol and also aids in relieving diverticulitis and preventing cancer of the lower bowel, it is best to begin using fiber gradually, by adding a little more each day until you are using 30 to 40 grams of dietary fiber daily. Cereal boxes and food packagings are a good source of information about dietary fiber. If the amount of fiber per serving isn't listed on the package, there probably isn't as much of it as you would like.

Dr. James D. Anderson, professor of medicine and clinical nutrition at the University of Kentucky and chief of the metabolic-endocrine section of the Veteran's Administrative Medical Center in Lexington, Kentucky, has pioneered new avenues of research using the High Carbohydrate High Fiber (HCF) Diet for diabetics and others. If you are interested in obtaining further information, you can write to HCF Nutrition Research Foundation, Inc., Box 22124, Lexington, Kentucky 40522.

The dietary-fiber content of some of the more common foods that are high in dietary fiber, based on work by Dr. Anderson and the U.S. Department of Agriculture, are shown in the following table.

DIETARY-FIBER CONTENT OF COMMON FOODS

Food	Grams of Dietary Fiber (rounded to nearest whole number)
FRUITS	
Apple, 1 medium	3
Apple juice, 1 cup	2
Applesauce, 1 cup	4
Apricots, fresh, 1 cup	4
Apricots, canned, 1 cup	7
Avocado, 1 medium	5
Banana, 1 medium	2
Blackberries, fresh, 1 cup	9
Blueberries, fresh, 1 cup	5
Boysenberries, fresh, 1 cup	11
Cherries, sour or sweet, canned or fresh, 1 cup	2
Cranberries, raw, 1 cup	4
Cranberries, cooked, 1 cup	8
Dates, dry, chopped, ½ cup	8
Fig, fresh, dried or canned, 1 medium	4
Fruit cocktail or salad, ½ cup	3
Grapefruit, fresh, ½ cup	2
Grapefruit, canned, ½ cup	1
Grapes, fresh, 12	1
Guava, fresh, 1 medium	5
Kiwi, fresh, 1 medium	1
Kumquat, fresh, 1 medium	1
Mango, raw, 1 cup cubes	1
Cantaloupe, fresh, 1 cup cubes	2

DIETARY-FIBER CONTENT OF COMMON FOODS

Food	Grams of Dietary Fiber (rounded to nearest whole number)
Casaba and honeydew melons, 1 cup cubes	1
Nectarine, fresh, 1 small	2
Orange, 1 small	2
Orange juice, 1 cup	1
Papaya, fresh, ⅓ medium	1
Passion fruit, 1 medium	6
Peach, fresh, 1 medium	2
Peaches, canned, 1 cup	4
Pear, fresh, 1 medium	5
Pears, canned, 1 cup	7
Pineapple, fresh or canned, 1 cup	2
Plums, fresh, 3 small	2
Purple plums, canned, 1 cup	5
Prunes, dried, 1 cup	21
Raisins, 1 cup	10
Raspberries, fresh or frozen, 1 cup	5
Rhubarb, fresh, 1 cup	3
Strawberries, fresh, 1 cup	4
Strawberries, sliced, 1 cup	4
Tangerine, fresh, 1 small	2

VEGETABLES

Food	Grams
Beans, ½ cup cooked	
Baby limas, dry limas, red, white, navy or pinto	5
Black-eyed, cowpeas, or chick-peas	12
Kidney	6
Bean sprouts, ½ cup	2
Beets, canned, ½ cup	2
Broccoli, fresh, ½ cup	3
Broccoli, cooked, ½ cup	2
Brussels sprouts, cooked, ½ cup	4
Cabbage, white, cooked, ½ cup	2
Cabbage, red, raw or cooked, ½ cup	1
Cabbage, white, raw, ½ cup	1
Carrots, raw, ½ cup	1

DIETARY-FIBER CONTENT OF COMMON FOODS

Food	Grams of Dietary Fiber (rounded to nearest whole number)
Carrots, cooked, ½ cup	2
Cauliflower, raw or cooked, ½ cup	2
Celery, raw or cooked, ½ cup	1
Chives, fresh, ½ cup	1
Collards, cooked, ½ cup	2
Corn, canned, whole kernel, ½ cup	6
Corn, canned, cream style, ½ cup	5
Corn, cooked, fresh, 1 medium ear	8
Cucumbers, raw, ½ cup	1
Eggplant, cooked, ½ cup	2
Endive or lettuce, fresh, 1 cup	1
Jerusalem artichoke, ½ cup	1
Leeks, fresh, ½ cup	2
Lentils, cooked, ½ cup	2
Mushrooms, raw, ½ cup	1
Mushrooms, cooked, ½ cup	2
Mustard greens, cooked, ½ cup	2
Okra, cooked, ½ cup	3
Onions, raw, ½ cup	3
Onions, cooked, ½ cup	2
Parsnips, cooked, ½ cup	3
Peas, green, raw or cooked, ½ cup	4
Peas, green, canned, ½ cup	8
Peas, green, frozen, cooked, ½ cup	5
Peas and carrots, cooked, ½ cup	5
Peppers, 1 medium	1
Potatoes	
White, cooked, peeled, escalloped, hashed brown, or mashed, ½ cup	2
White, baked with skin, 1 medium	4
Sweet, 1 medium	3
French-fried, 4 ounces	2
Chips, 2 ounces	1
Pumpkin, canned, ½ cup	4
Radishes, raw, red, 5 medium	1
Radishes, raw, white, 2 medium	1
Rutabagas, cooked, ½ cup	2
Sauerkraut, ½ cup	2

DIETARY-FIBER CONTENT OF COMMON FOODS

Food	Grams of Dietary Fiber (rounded to nearest whole number)
Spinach, raw, chopped, ½ cup	1
Spinach, cooked, ½ cup	3
Split peas, cooked, ½ cup	5
Squash, ½ cup	
Summer, cooked	1
Zucchini, raw	2
Zucchini, cooked	3
Winter, cooked	4
Tomatoes, fresh, 1 medium, ½ cup cooked, or ½ cup juice	1
Tomato sauce, canned, ½ cup	2
Tomato paste, canned, ½ cup	3
Turnips, cooked, ½ cup	2
Turnip greens, cooked, ½ cup	3
Turnip greens, canned, ½ cup	5
Vegetable juice cocktail, canned, ½ cup	1
Vegetables, mixed, canned, or frozen, ½ cup	2
Yam, cooked, ½ medium	3
Yam, raw, ½ cup	4
CEREAL (1 CUP)	
All Bran	26
Bran Buds	23
100% Bran	20
Corn Bran	8
Fiber One	24
Post's 40% Bran Flakes	7
Kellogg's 40% Bran Flakes	6
Raisin Bran	5
Grapenuts	9
Puffed Wheat	1
Shredded Wheat (1 rectangular biscuit) and Wheaties	3
Cream of Rice, cooked	5
Oat bran, cooked	9
Ralston and Roman Meal, cooked	4
Rolled Wheat, cooked	8

DIETARY-FIBER CONTENT OF COMMON FOODS

Food	Grams of Dietary Fiber (rounded to nearest whole number)
Whole Wheat Natural Cereal and Wheatena, cooked	3
Cream of Wheat and Oatmeal	2
FLOUR (1 CUP)	
All purpose, enriched	4
Bread and cake	3
Buckwheat	6
Corn and cornmeal	7
Rye	9
Soybean	12
Whole wheat, enriched	15
STARCHES (1 CUP)	
Bulgur, dry	12
Barley, pearled, dry	24
Rice, white enriched	
Cooked	Less than 1 gram
Raw	5
Rice, brown	
Cooked	5
Raw	14
Macaroni and noodles	
Dry	2
Cooked	1
BREADS (1 SLICE)	
Whole Bagels	1
Vienna, Pita, Pumpernickel, Raisin, and White	1
Cornbread	1
CRACKERS	
Graham, 2 squares	3
Saltines, 6	1
Whole Wheat, 5	2

6
EQUIPMENT AND INGREDIENTS

EQUIPMENT

Having and using the right equipment is a plus when you are preparing your low-cholesterol diabetic diet.

Knives

Sharp knives to prepare fruits and vegetables and to cut away all visible fat from meat and chicken are important—and I also like a good chopping knife and a knife with a serrated edge for slicing bread. One knife that has a specialized use is a rather round, thin, serrated knife, which is excellent for cutting fresh tomatoes. I don't use it for anything except slicing tomatoes but it is wonderful to have when I need it. A good boning knife and a knife for slicing are also important. If you have any doubt about the kinds of knives that you want, any good hardware store can recommend the types and kinds of knives that would be helpful for you.

Scales

I also find I need two different scales—a small one for weighing diabetic portions and a large one for weighing pounds and ounces when I'm cooking. I don't believe that diabetics should weigh everything they eat, but it is a good idea to weigh out portions occasionally to keep the feel of what is correct. So many times people will give themselves smaller portions than they are allowed because they think that something weighs more than it actually does.

Measuring Cups and Spoons

Standardized measuring cups and spoons are also essential. I like to keep several sets of measuring cups and spoons on hand so I can cook as I like without stopping to wash them. One set of measuring cups that I particularly like has ⅔-cup and ¾-cup measures in addition to the standard cup, ½-cup, ⅓-cup, and ¼-cup measures. Some sets have a coffee measure that holds 2 tablespoons and I find that very handy for measuring 2 tablespoons of an ingredient. Please don't ever use regular kitchen spoons for measuring. Most teaspoons hold about 1½ times the amount that measuring teaspoons hold and can wreak havoc with a cake or other baked item when substituted for a measuring spoon. Two-cup measures are also helpful, and I don't think I could do without my quart measure. If I have 2 cups of flour and some salt and baking powder as ingredients, I measure the flour in the quart measure up to the 2-cup line, and then add the salt and baking powder and stir it well before adding it to the other ingredients. Of course I also have the large glass measure for use in the microwave, and that also is a must—you can use it for so many things in the microwave as well as using it for measuring liquids.

Pots and Pans

There is such a variety of pots and pans that it is hard to recommend any one kind to the exclusion of the others. I like to use stainless steel for most of my pots and pans, although I don't know if I could get along without my cast iron skillets or my granite roaster. If you are happy with the ones you have now, there is no need to worry about changing; but if you feel you need new ones, I recommend heavy stainless steel of a good quality, particularly the ones with a layer of copper between two layers of stainless steel on the bottom of the pot. I keep a special pan for crèpes and blintzes, and of course have a large 3-gallon stainless steel pot for making soups and spaghetti sauce.

Casseroles

Casseroles are important and I use a variety of them—mostly Corning Ware and Pyrex, although there are some beautiful ones in enamelware these days. My friend Jessie Johnson was a home economist for Corning for many years and I have a rather complete set of Corning Ware because of her influence. Whenever something new came out and she told me about it, I generally went right out and bought it; I must say I've never been disappointed in any of it.

I like Corning Ware for refrigerator storage and use it a lot; but I also have a set of stainless steel refrigerator dishes with lids that are very handy, and I couldn't be without my stainless steel mixing bowls. My husband Chuck gave me the set of mixing bowls as an Easter gift the first year we were married. Though I thought it was a very unusual gift, they have been so handy that I wouldn't ever be without them now.

Thermometers

Two thermometers are helpful—a meat and a candy thermometer. I use the candy thermometer for checking the temperature of the liquid when I add yeast for bread. I suppose there may be a thermometer somewhere for bread-making; but if there is I've never seen it, and so I get along with my candy thermometer.

Mixers

One of my favorite pieces of equipment is my Kitchen Aid mixer. I have the largest size, which I think is best. Frances Nielsen has the middle size and she thinks that hers is the greatest, so I'm sure they are both wonderful. Several recipes in this book use the dough hook attachment on a mixer. If you don't have a dough hook on your mixer, use the mixer as long as you can and then pour the batter into a mixing bowl and do the rest of the bread mixing by hand. If you don't have a dough hook attachment for your mixer, I suggest you get one; you'll never be sorry that you did because it makes bread baking at home a cinch.

Food Processors

A food processor is also a big help. A low-cholesterol diabetic diet includes a lot of vegetables and fruits, and the food processor saves so much time preparing them that I don't know how we ever got along without one. I don't use it for a tablespoonful of chopped onions or other small quantities of food. However, I do use it to chop a cup or so of onions or celery to keep on hand in the refrigerator, because I use them so often.

Microwaves

I like to use a microwave oven to prepare vegetables. Most vegetables taste better, at least to us, when prepared in the microwave. You aren't losing a lot of vitamins and minerals in the water as you do when you cook the vegetables conventionally. I know that home economists and dietitians always tell you to save the vegetable cooking water for soups and sauces, but how many people actually bother to do that? I use the microwave oven to do so many things. I don't cook a lot of meat in it (although the makers say that you can) but I do use it to melt margarine, reheat foods, cook casseroles and vegetables, and bake apples and other fruits. I even use it to dehydrate parsley when Chuck has a good crop of it, and to dry bread when I want to make dry bread crumbs in a hurry. Since Chuck doesn't need to follow a diabetic diet, I cook some of my special foods in quantity and then reheat them a portion at a time when I want them—I like to be able to do that, also.

Chopping Boards

A good chopping board is a must. There are some very good plastic ones which don't dull the knife when you use them. They should be dishwasher-safe, easy to wipe off, and large enough to be efficient. I know that wooden chopping boards are hard to keep clean but sometimes they are worth it. I have a big bread board that Chuck made for his mother when he was taking woodworking in school; she used it for many years before I got it. It is such a help when I'm making bread, rolling out cookies, or shaping a coffee cake that I wouldn't be without it even if it is too big to fit into the dishwasher, and I do have to scrub it by hand whenever I use it.

Steamer

I like to use a stainless-steel steamer with a double boiler top and a steamer basket. Steamers help preserve vitamins and minerals in vegetables. Find a handy-sized one that will hold a bunch of broccoli or enough carrots for two meals (I like them hot the first meal and cold with diabetic dressing the second meal). It is best to get one that will steam only the amount of food you need. There is no sense using a big one and wasting the extra heat and water.

Dishwasher

I like my dishwasher, but the only way I can see in which it helps my diet is that it washes all of those dishes and pots and pans that I get dirty when I'm cooking. It really isn't essential—in fact I suppose it could be called a luxury—but I love it and intend to go right on using it. A friend of mine and I continue to argue over whether it is worthwhile or not. She insists that she can wash dishes in the same amount of time I spend cleaning off the table, getting the dishes ready for the dishwasher, and then putting them away. I'm afraid that it is an argument which will never be resolved—but we will go on being friends anyway.

Other Equipment

Of course I have all of the other usual equipment—spaghetti maker, toaster-oven, electric frying pan, etc.—but I try always to keep the use of equipment to a minimum in any cookbook I write. I feel that if you have specialized equipment and want to use it, you will know how to use it—and the recipe will still be practical for anyone who doesn't want to use any more equipment than necessary.

INGREDIENTS

It is important to understand which foods have cholesterol and which are cholesterol-free, as well as the cholesterol count of the foods that do contain cholesterol. The following table includes average cholesterol counts for various foods. The information is based on that found in the following references:

Nutritive Value of Foods. Home and Garden Bulletin no. 72. U.S. Department of Agriculture, Washington, D.C., 1981.

Composition of Foods, Raw, Processed, and Prepared. Agriculture Handbook no. 8. U.S. Department of Agriculture, Washington, D.C., 1963 and all current revisions.

INGREDIENTS

Item	Milligrams of cholesterol

DAIRY PRODUCTS

1 cup skim milk	4
1 cup buttermilk made from skim milk	4
1 cup whole milk	33
2 tablespoons sour cream	12
½ cup ice cream	29
½ cup soft-serve ice milk	7
½ cup sherbet	7
Cheese (per ounce)	
Cheddar	30
Colby	27
Cream	31
Mozzarella made with part skim milk	16
Parmesan	22
Ricotta made with skim milk	9
Swiss	24
Cheese spread	16
Cottage cheese	
½ cup creamed	16
½ cup uncreamed or dry	7
Neufchâtel	22

EGGS

1 egg yolk	272
1 egg white	0

FATS

1 tablespoon butter	31
¼ cup lard	49
1 tablespoon margarine made with vegetable oil	0
1 tablespoon vegetable oil	0

Item	Milligrams of cholesterol in 100 grams (about 3½ ounces) of lean meat, chicken, or fish
MEATS	
Lean beef	91
Light meat of chicken	58
Dark meat of chicken	80
Lamb	98
Pork, ham, fresh	68
Light meat of turkey	68
Dark meat of turkey	69
Veal, cutlet	128
Organ meats	
Beef brains, raw	1,672
Beef heart, raw	190
Beef kidney, raw	285
Beef liver, raw	354
Chicken liver	439
Beef sweetbreads, raw	223
FISH	
Cod, flounder, or halibut	43
Haddock	57
Pickled herring	13
Sockeye salmon, canned	44
Sardines in oil	142
Trout	58
Tuna, canned in water	42
Shellfish	
Clams and oysters, mixed species, raw	34
Crab, blue, raw	78
Lobster, northern, raw	95
Shrimp, mixed species, raw	152
MISCELLANEOUS	
Cereals	0
Vegetables	0
Fruit	0

I have discussed which foods are a plus and which shouldn't be used in the low-cholesterol diet at much greater length in Chapter 4, "Cholesterol."

Sugar Substitutes

Since we are all concerned about the use of sugar in our diabetic diets, I should explain that I have included a small amount of sugar in many of the recipes in this book. Most doctors and dietitians agree that some sugar may be used if it is calculated in the totals for the day. If you have any doubts about your own use of sugar, it would be wise to discuss this with your doctor before you use the recipes that contain sugar.

Most of us are accustomed to using sugar substitutes in our daily living. I hesitate to use tables because they always seem so dull but I think a table of sugar substitute equivalents might be helpful.

Sugar Substitute	Amount	Sugar Equivalent
Sprinkle Sweet and Sugar Twin	1 teaspoon	1 teaspoon
Sweet'n Low and Liquid Sucaryl	⅓ teaspoon 1 tablespoon	1 tablespoon ½ cup
Adolph's Sugar Substitute and Liquid Sweet 10	¼ teaspoon 1 tablespoon 4 teaspoons	1 tablespoon ¾ cup 1 cup
Weight Watchers	⅛ teaspoon 1 tablespoon	1 teaspoon ½ cup
Sweet-10 tablets and Equal tablets	1 tablet	1 teaspoon
Equal, granulated	1 packet	2 teaspoons

I use a variety of sugar substitutes when I am cooking. I like to use Equal (aspartame), but it can only be used to sweeten something that doesn't need to be cooked, so I keep Equal to sweeten things like soft drinks, gelatins, or fruits. If I think the sweetener should be combined with the dry ingredients, I generally use a dry sugar substitute, but if it should be mixed with the liquid ingredients, I use a liquid sugar substitute. I tend to use a little less sweetener than the makers recommend because I don't like an overwhelmingly sweet taste, but only you can decide how much you want to use. Use the amounts in this book as guides and decide how much you want in each recipe according to your own personal taste.

One thing to remember when using Equal is that it does have some nutritive value. One packet contains 4 calories and .96 grams of carbohydrate, so if you use several packets a day you have added that much carbohydrate to your intake for the day. The other sweeteners don't generally have any nutritive value and can be used as desired without counting them in your carbohydrate intake. However, none of the sweeteners add anything to the texture of baked items, so occasionally you need to use a little sugar or other sweetener for texture and browning.

Milk Products and Substitutes

Instant dry milk is also used frequently in these recipes. I have been using large quantities of instant dry milk for years. When I was working as a dietitian for the Army, one of the other dietitians in our department told me I should be known as "The Dry Milk Kid" because I was always preaching the value of dry milk. I wrote a small booklet on the proper use of dry milk, with recipes and methods in it, since I thought it was a good product and should be used whenever possible. I have also advocated its use in the nursing homes where I work as a dietary consultant. I was so pleased at a meeting to hear one of our dietary employees tell someone from another nursing home what a wonderful product dry milk is when it is used properly.

I like to use dry milk because it has all of the nutrients of whole milk except for the fat. It keeps well without refrigeration, is easy to store, is low in calories, and is less expensive than fresh milk. I have branched out over the last few years and now also use dry buttermilk because it is simpler to keep a can of dry buttermilk in the refrigerator than to keep liquid buttermilk on hand. I used to buy a quart of buttermilk, use a cup of it, and the rest would spoil—and then, too, it isn't always all that easy to buy low-fat buttermilk in our area. The regular instant dry milk whips easily with an equal measure of milk or fruit juice, partially set gelatin, or egg whites to add more variety to the diet.

Instant dry milk is particularly good in yeast breads—when using it you no longer need to scald the milk, it helps form a good brown crust, and it yields bread with a softer texture. Dry milk can be reconstituted and used as a beverage or in a recipe that needs liquid milk, or it can be used dry along with the flour or other ingredients.

Most packages of dry milk direct you to use ⅓ cup of instant dry milk to 1 cup of water. I use this as a regular measure, but you will find that some recipes in this book have only ¼ cup of instant dry milk to 1 cup of water. That is because when I am working on a diabetic recipe, I want to cut down on the carbohydrate as much as possible and therefore I use only as much of the milk as necessary to get good results.

Low-fat cottage cheese is usually available. If it isn't available, buy the regular cottage cheese and wash it off with lukewarm water to get rid of the cream, then put it back in the container with a little skim milk if you like it creamy.

If you are accustomed to using cream in your coffee, you can use instant dry milk or one of the coffee whiteners which list a vegetable oil as their main ingredient. Be careful not to buy a coffee whitener that includes palm oil, coconut oil, or hydrogenated vegetable oil as an ingredient. Better yet, drink your coffee black—or best of all, stop drinking coffee. Tests and research seem to be telling us that coffee isn't all that good for us.

Vegetable Oils and Margarine

Learning to use vegetable oil instead of lard, bacon fat, butter, or shortening seems to be one of the hardest things for most cooks to do when they start on a low-cholesterol diet. One way to convince yourself that it is a good idea is to remind yourself that with solid fats, you have to melt the fat you are using before you fry anything; but with oil, you are starting out with the fat already "melted." I discovered when I started counting fat exchanges for my diabetic diet that I didn't really need to use all of that oil in the bottom of a frying pan for frying foods. One or two tablespoons of vegetable oil in the bottom of a pan heated to frying temperature is sufficient to cook most meats or vegetables, and the vegetable oil doesn't burn and turn brown as easily as butter.

The type of fat used makes a difference in the texture and flavor of baked goods. You can generally substitute margarine for butter on an equal basis. You can use vegetable oil to substitute for melted fat in recipes, but if the original recipe specified shortening or butter, you will get better results using margarine. Oil can sometimes be substituted for softened butter or shortening, but if the basic recipe that you are trying to change creams the butter and sugar together, it is best to use margarine in the recipe.

Vegetable oil should be kept in a cool spot, out of sunlight, because you don't want it to get rancid. It shouldn't be refrigerated unless it won't be used for a long time, but too high a temperature will also be harmful. I keep my reserve supply in the fruit room in the basement and oil that I am using every day in the kitchen.

It is always a good idea to read the ingredient list of any item; it is particularly important when you are buying margarine. You need to know what kind of fat has been used in the margarine. Vegetable oil should be the first ingredient in a margarine acceptable on a low-cholesterol diet and you don't even want to consider a margarine that contains lard or animal fat. If you are in doubt about your local brands, call your Heart Association and ask them to recommend the best ones in your area—and remember, a fat exchange is a fat exchange no matter what brand of margarine you use.

Eggs and Egg Substitutes

Liquid egg substitute is based on egg whites and is a wonderful substitute for whole eggs. It is more expensive than egg whites so I try to use egg whites whenever possible; however, there are certain recipes that need whole eggs and liquid egg substitute works very well when you aren't supposed to be using egg yolks.

People often ask me what to do with leftover egg yolks that aren't used. I freeze mine with 1 teaspoon of salt or 2 teaspoons of sugar per cup and give them to Frances Nielsen whose family doesn't have any problem with cholesterol. At first it was difficult for me to throw away egg yolks, but now I find myself doing it often when I have only one or two yolks. I tell myself how wonderful it is that I can so easily dispose of all that cholesterol without worrying about it and just toss it down the garbage disposal. If you like, you can buy dehydrated egg whites and then you won't have to toss away the yolks. It costs about the same over a period of time.

Oat Bran

Oat bran has proved to be a very valuable source of water-soluble fiber, which helps reduce both blood sugar and cholesterol in the blood. I am convinced that oat bran should be a part of every diabetic's diet. I have included several recipes using oat bran in this first revision, and I hope you will use them. We use oat bran as a breakfast cereal, but since we don't like it plain, we use one half oat bran and one half oatmeal and then cook it as we would oatmeal. (We use twice as much water as cereal. Bring the water to a boil; add the cereal; cook while stirring constantly for 1 minute; remove from heat and let sit, covered, for 5 minutes; then serve hot with skim milk and sugar substitute.) Oat bran can be purchased in bulk or packages at a health food store. It is also available in one-pound packages like other hot cereals or in bags at most grocery stores. I have found that you can use half oat bran and half all-purpose flour in most hot bread recipes. That way you can add it to your own favorite recipes with good results. It is very good in cookies, although we don't get many of them, and again can be substituted for half of the oatmeal in oatmeal cookies or half of the flour in other types of cookies. I keep a canister of oat bran with my other baking ingredients, but I keep my reserve supply in the freezer to keep it fresh as I would other flours. It has fewer calories than flour and adds a lot of fiber to your recipes.

I've known several people who brought their cholesterol level down and helped control their blood sugar with oat bran. I try to always have a supply of oat-bran muffins in the freezer so that I can eat at least two of them every day in addition to my cereal.

Other Ingredients

There is only one ingredient used in this book that doesn't fit into a low-cholesterol diabetic diet. All of the other ingredients are acceptable on the diet, but I did include a recipe for chocolate chip cookies. There isn't that much cholesterol in the chips, and they can be fit into the typical doctor-recommended limit of 300 milligrams of cholesterol per day—so I used them. After all, chocolate chip cookies are a part of the American way—we would hate to have to get along without them completely!

If you have a question about some ingredient that I haven't used in a recipe, check the tables of nutritive values in Chapter 2, "Calculating Food Exchanges," and if the ingredient is listed you will know that it is acceptable in your diet.

Fruits, vegetables, and cereals are all free of cholesterol and are mostly complex carbohydrates that are recognized to be good for us. Vegetables and fruits should be used as much as possible because they are high in fiber and most of them are low in carbohydrates. A vegetable plate has most of the nutrients we need for a well-balanced meal along with a little cottage cheese, lean meat, or fish.

Since fiber is so good for us, I have used oat bran, whole wheat flour, and other whole grains as often as possible in these recipes. Whole wheat flour and graham flour have the same nutrients except that graham flour has been ground to yield a finer texture and therefore is more suitable in some recipes.

Bread flour is also used several times. Bread flour has a higher gluten content than all-purpose flour and helps make really good bread. It takes more liquid than all-purpose flour, but the final product has a finer texture and greater strength.

Since you will no longer be buying commercial mixes because of the fat and sugar in them, you can make your own or mix up a fresh batch each time. Angel food cake mix or mixes to which you add the egg and fat are acceptable if you add oil and liquid egg substitute to them; however, beware of using most mixes because they usually have ingredients that you shouldn't use.

Cocoa is used in these recipes instead of chocolate because chocolate contains cocoa butter, which isn't good on a low-cholesterol diet. Three tablespoons of cocoa plus one tablespoon of fat is equal to 1 ounce of baking chocolate. The cocoa can also be mixed with boiling water without any fat, and used as a chocolate substitute with very good results. (Use only enough boiling water to make a smooth paste.)

Low-sodium variations are included for the recipes whenever practical. I haven't stressed using salt substitutes because not all doctors approve of them for all patients. If you want to use them, it is best to discuss them with your doctor. Each patient is different and no doctor will make a blanket statement that everyone can use salt substitutes.

The low-sodium diet notes in these recipes are planned for low-sodium diets, not salt-free diets. I discussed these variations with Mary Agnes Jones, R.D., of Holy Cross Hospital in Chicago and with Muriel Urbashich, R.D., head of the dietary department of South Chicago Community Hospital. They both agreed that the low-sodium diet is more liberal than it used to be. Therefore I have used regular milk on the low-sodium diet, rather than salt-free milk. Salt-free margarine is available in most stores now and several packagers are now offering low-sodium canned vegetables that also may be used. Low-sodium soups are also available. Anyone on a "no added salt" diet can use the basic recipes in this book by deleting the salt when salt is specified. Some recipes that contain soy sauce or other highly salted ingredients cannot be changed successfully so they are not recommended for use on a low-sodium diet.

Ice milk, fruit ices, and sherbet can be used on the low-cholesterol diet, so feel free to use them within the limits of your diabetic diet.

The most important thing to remember when planning your low-cholesterol diabetic diet is that you have many food items left that you can use. It is best to work with those and see what interesting and tasty dishes you can develop rather than mourning the loss of those few foods that are no longer available to you.

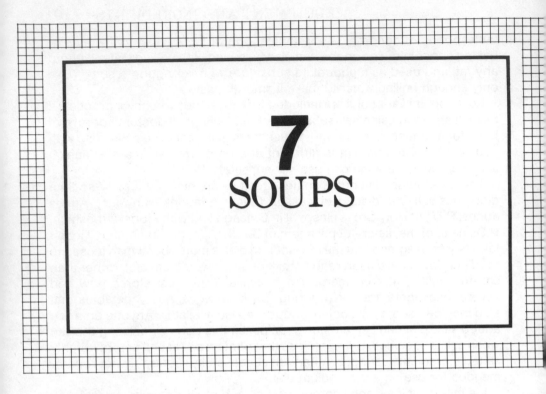

7
SOUPS

Soup is always a good addition to a low-cholesterol diabetic diet. For the diabetic diet you are interested only in the amount of carbohydrate, protein, and fat in the soup; however, for the low-cholesterol diet you also want to substitute polyunsaturated fats for animal fats, so you need to find substitutes for the animal fat, egg yolks, cream, whole milk, or butter often used in soup recipes.

There are all sorts of tricks you can use to change a high-cholesterol soup into one suitable for a low-cholesterol diet. Liquid egg substitute can be used instead of egg yolks, margarine or oil instead of butter, a double amount of instant dry milk instead of evaporated milk, and a little more margarine in the soup along with the milk instead of cream. Of course this changes the flavor a little bit (but not too much) and the soups are still good in their own right.

I would have liked to have been able to include more soups in this chapter based on dried peas, beans, and lentils. I wasn't able to include too many of them, since they are so high in carbohydrate that one bowl of soup takes up most of a meal's allowance. Therefore, I concentrated on vegetable soups that provide fiber with less carbohydrate.

Because many soups are based on a good, rich chicken or beef broth, and because a low-cholesterol diet needs broth without any animal fat in it, I use a great deal of the fat-free chicken and beef broth concentrates available in the stores. These concentrates generally have a large amount of salt in them so the sodium count is very high when they are used. If you are on a low-sodium diet, you can handle this by buying low-sodium bouillon cubes or by preparing your own low-sodium, fat-free broth. When buying low-sodium soup concentrates, check the list of ingredients carefully, because several of them are based on animal fats instead of salt, which aren't acceptable on a low-cholesterol diet.

If you decide to make your own low-sodium, fat-free broth, start by buying (if you don't have one) a heavy stainless steel or aluminum stock pot with a 2- or 3-gallon capacity and a tight-fitting lid. The broth needs to cook for a long time to develop flavor and it isn't worth doing unless you can cook a large amount. The broth freezes well and can be frozen in containers holding the right amount for future soups or casseroles. I have a heavy stainless steel 3-gallon pot that I bought when we were first married. I couldn't count the amount of soup, spaghetti sauce, and other things that I have cooked in that pot and it still looks as bright and shiny as it did the day we bought it.

I used very little salt in most of the soup recipes containing broth because I used the commercial bouillon cubes that are high in salt in making the broth. If you use your own broth you will probably have to add salt (if you can) or a salt substitute if your doctor approves.

FAT-FREE, LOW-SODIUM BEEF BROTH

Although we class it as beef broth, veal bones are also very good and may be used whenever available. I don't care for lamb or pork bones in broth although the British do make a lamb broth that they prize very much.

Any beef or veal bones are acceptable. You can get soup bones or soup meat from your butcher, save any bones from roasts, and collect any available bones from your family until you have enough to make a good, big pot of broth. It just isn't worthwhile unless you save enough bones.

Beef or veal bones, any kind
1 onion
2 carrots
1–2 celery stalks
Water to cover, at room temperature

The broth will have a better flavor if you roast the bones and trimmings in an open roaster in the oven at 350° F. until they are well browned. This helps develop the flavor of the broth. Cool the bones to room temperature, place in a stock pot, and cover with onion, a couple of carrots, and a stalk or so of celery at this time. Cover and simmer for 4–6 hours. Scum will rise to the top when the liquid first begins to simmer and it is a good idea to skim most of this off. (It is almost impossible to get it all off; I know, I've tried it often enough.) The broth may look done to you long before the cooking time is ended, but it won't have the flavor and body it will have if cooked the full length of time.

Remove from heat. Strain well, putting the broth in a pan and leaving the bones out. Refrigerate the broth until the fat has risen to the top and solidified. Remove the fat, place the clear broth in another container, and freeze or refrigerate until needed. At this stage I add any broth, with the fat removed, that I have gathered from roasts. The broth from the roasts also has a good flavor and seems to add something to the broth. (Throw away the murky part at the bottom of the broth.)

As soon as the bones are cool enough to handle, remove any meat from them and refrigerate or freeze until needed. This meat is excellent for future use in soups. Discard the bones and any bits of overcooked vegetables with them.

Since this broth is considered free on a diabetic diet, it may be used for soups or other uses without adding any nutritive values that need to be counted.

FAT-FREE, LOW-SODIUM CHICKEN OR TURKEY BROTH

Chicken or turkey bones, necks, wings
1 onion
2 carrots, small
2 celery stalks
A little parsley
1 quart cold water for each pound of bones

Weigh the chicken or turkey bones, necks, and wings, place in a stock pot, and add 1 quart cold water for each pound of bones. Don't add any giblets, skin, or fat because they are all forbidden on a low-cholesterol diet. Bring the water to a boil, reduce heat, and simmer 5 minutes. Drain well. Replace with the same amount of cold water. Add 1 onion, 2 small carrots, a couple of stalks of celery, and a little parsley. Cover tightly and simmer for 2½–3 hours. If you are using a precooked carcass of a turkey or chicken with no raw bones, it isn't necessary to discard the first liquid. Just cover with cold water and simmer an hour or so or until the meat is falling off the bones. If the carcass is still whole, you will get a richer broth if you crush the bones or separate them so they won't need as much water to cover them.

After the cooking period, strain the broth, setting aside the chicken or turkey bones to cool. Chill the broth until the fat has risen to the top and solidified. Discard the fat. Remove the clear broth to another container and freeze or refrigerate until used. (Throw away the murky part at the bottom of the pot.)

Pick any chicken or turkey meat off the bones as soon as they are cool enough to handle and refrigerate or freeze it for future use in soups, discarding the bones.

Since this broth is considered free on a diabetic diet, it may be used for soups or other uses without adding any nutritive values that need to be counted.

BARLEY MUSHROOM SOUP

Yields 3 quarts—12 servings

"Chef Dave" Hutchins gave me this recipe. It is kosher as long as you use vegetable stock, which you can buy in a health food store or some supermarkets. I'm happy to say that Chef Dave is very careful to follow low-cholesterol guidelines when cooking or planning food for his restaurant, Johnson's Supper Club, in Elkader, Iowa. This low-cholesterol food is greatly appreciated by his many older patrons who are attempting to keep their cholesterol count under 200.

¾ **cup pearl barley**
¼ **cup vegetable oil**
2 pounds sliced fresh mushrooms
2 cups diced celery
2 cups julienne onions
4 minced garlic cloves
3 quarts vegetable stock
Salt to taste
⅛ **to ¼ teaspoon freshly ground black pepper**
½ **cup plain yogurt**
¼ **cup mushroom-flavored or regular soy sauce**

Put barley in a food processor, preferably a small one, and give it a couple of pulses to chop barley into grits. Set aside.

Preheat a 4- or 6-quart heavy pot on medium heat for 1 minute. Swirl oil around the bottom of pot. Add mushrooms and cook, stirring frequently, until mushrooms are well browned. Add celery, onions, and garlic and continue to cook and stir until onions are soft. Add vegetable stock and barley and bring to a rolling boil. (If you don't have vegetable stock, you can use fat-free beef stock, in which case the soup will no longer be kosher). Decrease heat, cover, and simmer until barley is tender. Add salt and pepper (the amount of salt you need will depend upon the saltiness of the stock).

Remove soup from heat and stir ½ cup of it into yogurt. Add yogurt mixture and soy sauce to soup. Serve hot, but don't boil after adding yogurt. Use 1 cup per serving.

Nutritive values per serving:

CAL	CHO (gm)	PRO (gm)	FAT (gm)	NA (mg)
129	17	5	5	1427 (without added salt)

Food exchanges per serving:
Low-sodium diets:

1 broad, 1 fat
Omit salt and use low-sodium vegetable or beef broth.

CABBAGE AND RICE SOUP

Yields 2 quarts—8 servings

1 tablespoon vegetable oil
1 pound (about 5 cups) shredded cabbage
1 cup thinly sliced onions
4 cups fat-free beef broth
4 cups fat-free chicken broth
Sprinkle of pepper
¼ teaspoon grated nutmeg
½ cup long-grain rice

Preheat a heavy saucepan on medium heat for 1 minute. Swirl oil around bottom of pan. Add cabbage and onions and cook, stirring frequently, over medium heat until cabbage and onions are soft. Add broths, pepper, nutmeg, and rice. Cover and simmer about 20 minutes, or until rice is tender. Do not overcook. Serve hot, using 1 cup soup per serving.

Nutritive values per serving:

CAL	CHO (gm)	PRO (gm)	FAT (gm)	NA (mg)
81	14	3	2	969

Food exchanges per serving:
Low-sodium diets:

1 bread
Omit salt-free broths.

CHUNKY SPLIT PEA SOUP

Yields 6 cups—8 servings

This soup has little bits of vegetable in it. If you want a smoother soup, it can be puréed in the blender or food processor before it is served.

1 cup dried split peas
6 cups water
6 chicken bouillon cubes
1 cup finely chopped onions
¼ cup finely chopped celery
¼ cup finely chopped fresh green peppers
¼ cup finely chopped fresh carrots
2 tablespoons margarine
¼ teaspoon ground thyme
Salt and pepper to taste

Wash split peas and put in a saucepan. Add water and bouillon cubes; cover and simmer 1½ hours, stirring frequently.

Add onions, celery, peppers, and carrots to split peas; cover and simmer ½ hour, stirring frequently.

Add margarine and seasonings to soup and continue to simmer for 10 minutes. Remove from heat and serve hot. Serve ¾ cup per serving. (The amount of salt needed will depend upon the saltiness of the bouillon cubes. The recipe is calculated using chicken bouillon cubes instead of salt-free chicken broth.)

Nutritive values per serving:	CAL	CHO (gm)	PRO (gm)	FAT (gm)	NA (mg)
	128	19	7	3	774

Food exchanges per serving: 1 bread, 1 lean meat

Low-sodium diets: Use low-sodium broth instead of the water and chicken bouillon cubes, or delete chicken bouillon cubes and use only water. Use salt-free margarine and don't add any salt to the soup.

CREAM OF TOMATO SOUP

Yields about 4 cups—6 servings

This recipe is from Vera Wilson, a friend of mine from here in Wadena. She makes it with home-canned tomato juice, but it is also good made with commercially canned tomato juice.

1 tablespoon finely chopped onion
3 tablespoons margarine
3 tablespoons all-purpose flour
1 teaspoon salt
⅛ teaspoon pepper
2 cups tomato juice
2 cups milk at room temperature
1 1-gram packet Equal (aspartame) sugar substitute

Fry onions in margarine in a saucepan, stirring constantly, until soft but not brown. Add flour and seasonings to onions and cook and stir over moderate heat until bubbly but not browned.

Add tomato juice to flour mixture. Bring to a boil, stirring constantly, for 1 minute. Stir tomato mixture into milk. Place soup in the top of a double boiler. Return to heat and heat to serving temperature. Remove from heat.

Stir Equal into soup and serve hot, ¾ cup per serving.

Nutritive values per serving:	CAL	CHO (gm)	PRO (gm)	FAT (gm)	NA (mg)
	111	11	4	6	630

Food exchanges per serving: 1 milk, 1 fat

Low-sodium diets: Omit salt. Use salt-free margarine and tomato juice canned without salt.

GOULASH SOUP

Yields 2 quarts—8 servings

*Muriel Urbashich, the dietitian who is the head of the Dietary Depart-
ment at South Chicago Community Hospital, tells me that this soup is a
great favorite in their employees' cafeteria. They sell gallons of it whenever
they have it on the menu. Muriel and I have done three large-quantity
cookbooks together and spend a lot of time talking recipes and food
preparation when we get together.*

2 cups chopped onions
3 tablespoons vegetable oil
1 pound beef round
8 cups fat-free broth
¼ teaspoon garlic powder
2 teaspoons paprika
½ cup drained, crushed, canned tomatoes
Salt to taste
1½ cups diced fresh white potatoes

Brown onions in 2 tablespoons vegetable oil in a heavy frying pan over
moderate heat, stirring occasionally. Transfer onions with a slotted spoon to
a heavy saucepan.

Add remaining tablespoon of oil to frying pan. Trim all visible fat from the
beef and cut it into ¾-inch cubes. (This is easier if the meat is slightly
frozen.) Brown beef in the frying pan over moderate heat, stirring occasionally. Transfer meat with a slotted spoon into saucepan with the onions.
Discard as much fat as possible from the frying pan.

Add broth to frying pan and cook and stir over low heat to get as many of
the brown particles in the pan as possible into the broth. Pour the hot broth
into the saucepan with the onions and meat.

Add seasonings and tomatoes to meat and broth. Cover and simmer over
low heat until meat is tender. Remove from heat. Cool to room temperature.
Refrigerate until thoroughly chilled and the fat has risen to the top. Remove
the fat and discard it. Return the soup to heat. Taste for seasoning and add
salt, if necessary.

Add potatoes to soup. Cover and simmer 15–20 minutes or until the
potatoes are tender. Serve 1 cup hot soup per serving.

Nutritive values per serving:	CAL	CHO (gm)	PRO (gm)	FAT (gm)	NA (mg)
	95	9	13	negl.	1,023

Food exchanges per serving: 2 lean meat, ½ bread

Low-sodium diets: Use low-sodium broth and fresh tomatoes or tomatoes canned without salt.

GAZPACHO

Yields about 4½ cups—6 servings

This is refreshing on a warm summer day—a good way to celebrate the first ripe tomatoes in summer, although it is equally tasty later in the fall.

3 cups fat-free beef broth
¾ cup tomato juice
2 tablespoons lemon juice
3 tablespoons Spicy Tomato Dressing (see index)
⅓ cup finely chopped onions
⅓ cup finely chopped fresh green peppers
2 tablespoons finely chopped celery
1 cup diced, peeled, and cored fresh tomatoes
¼ teaspoon garlic powder
1 teaspoon salt
1 tablespoon chopped parsley
¼–½ cup thinly sliced or diced cucumbers

Combine all ingredients except cucumbers; mix lightly and refrigerate overnight or at least 4 hours.

Serve soup in chilled cups garnished with cucumbers, using ¾ cup soup per serving.

Nutritive values per serving:	CAL	CHO (gm)	PRO (gm)	FAT (gm)	NA (mg)
	35	5	1	1	944

Food exchanges per serving: 1 vegetable

Low-sodium diets: Omit salt. Use low-sodium broth and the low-sodium variation of the salad dressing.

FRUIT SOUP

Yields 6 cups—12 servings

I can never decide if this is a soup or a fruit. I generally serve it as a dessert, so I calculated it using a ½-cup serving. If you want to serve it chilled or hot as a soup, it would be 2 fruit exchanges for a 1-cup portion.

4 cups water
2 whole cinnamon sticks
1 teaspoon whole cloves
3 tablespoons instant tapioca
⅓ cup white raisins
1 cup drained, canned unsweetened mandarin oranges
1 cup drained, canned unsweetened pineapple tidbits
1 cup drained, canned unsweetened diced peaches
Sugar substitute equal to ⅔ cup sugar

Combine water, cinnamon, and cloves in a saucepan. Cover and bring to a boil. Reduce heat and simmer for 5 minutes. Remove from heat and allow to marinate overnight. Drain spices from the liquid and discard spices.

Add tapioca and raisins to liquid and let stand at room temperature for 5 minutes. Place in saucepan, cover, and simmer until clear. Remove from heat.

Add fruits and sweetener to soup and refrigerate at least overnight before serving. If you want to serve it warm, it can be reheated after it has marinated. Serve ½ cup per serving.

Nutritive values per serving:	CAL	CHO (gm)	PRO (gm)	FAT (gm)	NA (mg)
	41	11	negl.	negl.	3

Food exchanges per serving: 1 fruit
Low-sodium diets: May be served as written.

GOLDEN SQUASH SOUP

Yields 2 quarts—8 servings

This recipe is a memento of my trip to Argentina. They use squash much more frequently than we do as a vegetable as well as in soups and stews. I loved their food, but I never did get used to having dinner at ten o'clock in the evening.

2 tablespoons margarine
¾ cup finely chopped onion
⅓ cup all-purpose flour
½ cup instant dry milk
2 cups hot water
6 cups fat-free chicken broth at room temperature
2 cups cooked, puréed winter squash
⅛ teaspoon white pepper
½ teaspoon celery salt
¼ to 1 teaspoon curry powder
½ teaspoon salt
2 tablespoons chopped chives or parsley

Preheat a heavy saucepan over medium heat for 1 minute. Melt margarine in pan, add onions, and cook and stir over medium heat until onions are soft and lightly browned. Sprinkle flour evenly over onions and continue to cook and stir until flour is lightly browned. Dissolve milk in hot water, combine with broth (combined liquid should be lukewarm), and add to onions and flour. Cook and stir over medium heat until smooth and thickened. Add puréed squash, pepper, celery salt, curry powder, and salt. Simmer 5 minutes. Serve hot, garnished with chives or parsley, using 1 cup soup per serving.

Nutritive values per serving:	CAL	CHO (gm)	PRO (gm)	FAT (gm)	NA (mg)
	107	14	5	3	911

Food exchanges per serving: 1 bread, ½ fat
Low-sodium diets: Use salt-free broths and omit salt.

MINESTRONE SOUP

Yields 3 quarts—12 servings

This is a hearty Italian vegetable soup that is high in fiber. I think it is my favorite soup. I generally make a double batch and freeze most of it in containers to use later. It is high in sodium because I calculated it with commercial beef concentrate for the beef broth. If you are watching your salt, you should prepare it with homemade or low-sodium beef broth. Most minestrone contains pasta in some form but I leave that out because I want to use my bread exchanges for crackers with my soup.

3 quarts fat-free beef broth
1 cup peeled, diced fresh white potatoes
½ cup chopped onions
½ cup chopped carrots
¼ cup diced celery
¼ cup diced fresh green peppers
1 tablespoon chopped parsley
1 cup diced canned tomatoes and juice
½ cup coarsely chopped cabbage
2 cups (16-ounce can) cooked navy or great northern beans
½ teaspoon garlic powder
Salt to taste
¼ teaspoon pepper
1½ teaspoons Italian seasoning
1 teaspoon leaf oregano
½ teaspoon basil
1½ cups diced cooked beef without visible fat
Water as necessary

Place first six ingredients in a large soup kettle, at least 6 quarts; cover and simmer for 15 minutes.

Add all remaining ingredients except meat to soup, cover, and simmer for another 15 minutes.

Add meat to soup. Add enough water, if necessary, to make 3 quarts soup. Serve hot, 1 cup per serving.

Nutritive values per serving:

CAL	CHO (gm)	PRO (gm)	FAT (gm)	NA (mg)
101	11	10	2	996

Food exchanges per serving: 2 vegetable, 1 lean meat
Low-sodium diets: Use salt-free broth. Add salt substitute to taste instead of salt to taste.

TOMATO BOUILLON

Yields 2 quarts—10 servings

1 cup chopped celery
1 cup chopped onions
2 cups fat-free chicken broth
3 cups fat-free beef broth
3 cups tomato juice
1 teaspoon Worcestershire sauce
¼ teaspoon basil
Whisper of black pepper

Place celery, onions, and chicken broth in saucepan. Cover and simmer 30 minutes. Drain well. Discard vegetables and return broth to saucepan.

Add beef broth, tomato juice, and seasonings to chicken broth. Cover and simmer for about 5 minutes. Taste for seasoning and add more, if necessary. Serve ¾ cup hot or cold bouillon per serving.

Nutritive values per serving:

CAL	CHO (gm)	PRO (gm)	FAT (gm)	NA (mg)
17	3	1	negl.	633

Food exchanges per serving: 1 serving may be considered free.
Low-sodium diets: Use low-sodium broths and tomato juice. Delete Worcestershire sauce and add ¼ teaspoon ground thyme or leaf oregano.

GREEN AND GOLD CREAM SOUP

Yields 4 cups—6 servings

This is a basic cream soup. Other vegetables in the same vegetable food group may be substituted for the carrots and broccoli. The vegetables may also be puréed before they are added to the soup—but I like the small bits of vegetables in the soup.

1 cup frozen or fresh broccoli stems and pieces
1 cup finely chopped carrots
3 tablespoons flour
2 tablespoons margarine
4 cups fat-free chicken broth
2 tablespoons instant dry milk
¼ teaspoon salt

Chop broccoli into small pieces. They should be large enough to have a little texture but not very large. Place in a small container, cover, and cook for 2 minutes on high in the microwave or cook until barely tender in a small amount of water. Drain well and set aside.

Place carrots in a small container. Add 1 tablespoon water, cover, and cook on high in the microwave for 6–8 minutes or until tender, or cook until barely tender in a small amount of water. Drain well and set aside.

Place flour and margarine in a 1½- or 2-quart saucepan over moderate heat. Cook and stir until smooth. Stir broth, dry milk, and salt together and add to flour mixture. Cook and stir over moderate heat until smooth and thickened. Continue to cook, stirring frequently, over low heat for 1 more minute. Add vegetables and reheat to serving temperature. Serve ¾ cup soup per serving.

Nutritive values per serving:	CAL	CHO (gm)	PRO (gm)	FAT (gm)	NA (mg)
	71	7	2	4	795

Food exchanges per serving: 1 fat, ½ bread
Low-sodium diets: Omit salt. Use salt-free margarine and low-sodium broth.

POTAGE PIERRE

Yields 10½ cups—7 servings

This luscious soup is from Beverly Wolfrum of Aurora, Colorado. She and I share a crusading fervor aimed at helping people lower their cholesterol counts. She told me she has been using this recipe since her husband was a seminarian and she needed to use economical recipes. Don't change a thing in this recipe; it is wonderful just as it is written. You may think it is ready after 2 hours, but please simmer it for at least 4 hours because the flavor continues to improve.

1 pound lean beef with fat and gristle removed
1 29-ounce can whole tomatoes and juice
¾ cup finely chopped onions
¾ cup finely chopped celery
¾ cup finely chopped carrots
4 cups fat-free beef broth
1 teaspoon thyme
10 whole peppercorns

Place meat in a 4-quart pot. Chop tomatoes and add with their juice to meat. Add onions, celery, carrots, broth, thyme, and peppercorns. Cover and simmer 4 to 5 hours. Add hot water if necessary to keep yield at 10½ cups. Serve hot, using 1½ cups per serving.

Nutritive values per serving:	CAL	CHO (gm)	PRO (gm)	FAT (gm)	NA (mg)
	119	8	15	3	987

Food exchanges per serving: 2 vegetable, 2 lean meat
Low-sodium diets: Use low-sodium canned tomatoes and salt-free broth.

MULLIGATAWNY SOUP

Yields 7 cups—7 servings

This soup is delicious and I think it is well worth the bread exchange it costs me.

¼ **cup chopped onions**
¼ **cup chopped fresh green pepper**
¼ **cup diced celery**
2 **tablespoons vegetable oil**
⅓ **cup flour**
5 **cups fat-free chicken broth at room temperature**
1 **small (4 to the pound) tart apple**
¾ **cup drained, crushed canned tomatoes**
¼ **teaspoon curry powder**
⅛ **teaspoon ground cloves**
Whisper of white pepper
1 **cup diced cooked chicken with fat and skin removed**
1 **cup cooked rice**

Fry onions, pepper, and celery in oil in a heavy saucepan over moderate heat, stirring frequently, until the onions are limp but not browned. Remove vegetables from the pan with a slotted spoon and reserve for later use.

Add flour to oil in pan and cook and stir over moderate heat until smooth and lightly browned. Add broth to flour mixture and cook and stir over moderate heat until thickened. Add the reserved vegetables.

Wash and core apple and cut into small pieces as though you were going to make Waldorf salad. Add to soup. Add tomatoes and seasonings to soup. Cover and simmer for 45 minutes or until the vegetables are tender.

Add chicken and rice to the soup just before it is served. Reheat soup if necessary and serve 1 cup hot soup per serving.

Nutritive values per serving:	CAL	CHO (gm)	PRO (gm)	FAT (gm)	NA (mg)
	135	14	8	5	836

Food exchanges per serving: 1 bread, 1 lean meat
Low-sodium diets: Use low-sodium broth and rice cooked without salt.

SWISS SOUP

Yields 7 cups—7 servings

I like having a soup that I can eat without counting it as a food exchange. It is a good pick me up in the afternoon or late evening if I'm hungry and tired of munching on celery. You can place 1-2 ounces of lean, cubed cooked beef in a soup bowl and add this soup for a good vegetable-beef soup which only costs you the meat exchanges.

1 tablespoon margarine
¼ cup chopped onions
½ cup chopped celery
¼ cup chopped carrots
¼ cup chopped fresh green peppers
6 cups fat-free beef broth
2 cups shredded cabbage
¹⁄₁₆ teaspoon black pepper (optional)
Salt to taste
¼ teaspoon ground nutmeg

Melt the margarine in the bottom of a saucepan. Add onions, celery, carrots, and peppers and cook and stir over moderate heat about 4 minutes or until the vegetables are limp but not browned.

Add broth to vegetables; cover and simmer 15 minutes.

Add cabbage and seasonings to soup. Cover and simmer another 5 minutes. Serve soup hot, 1 cup per serving.

Nutritive values per serving:	CAL	CHO (gm)	PRO (gm)	FAT (gm)	NA (mg)
	30	3	1	2	449*
Food exchanges per serving:	1 cup may be considered free.				
Low-sodium diets:	Do not add salt. Use salt-free margarine.				

*without adding salt

VEGETABLE BEEF SOUP

Yields 2 quarts—8 servings

1½ pounds beef stew meat
Cold water as necessary
2 quarts cold water
1½ teaspoons salt
⅛ teaspoon black pepper
1 cup diced fresh white potatoes
½ cup diced carrots
1 cup coarsely chopped onions
½ cup shredded cabbage
1 cup canned tomatoes and juice
½ cup fresh or frozen green string beans cut into ½-inch pieces

Trim any gristle and visible fat from meat with a sharp knife. Place meat in a saucepan. Cover with cold water, bring to a boil, and boil 1 minute. Remove meat from broth and discard broth. Return meat to saucepan.

Add 2 quarts cold water, salt, and pepper to meat. Bring to a boil. Reduce heat, cover, and simmer for about 1½ hours or until meat is tender. Drain the broth from the meat. Strain the broth, cover, and refrigerate meat and broth separately. After the broth is chilled, remove the hard fat from the top of the broth.

Measure the broth and add cold water to the broth to equal 7 cups of liquid. Add vegetables to stock. Cover and simmer 30–45 minutes or until vegetables are tender. Taste for seasoning and add more if desired. (Nutritive values are calculated using 1½ teaspoons salt.) Add meat to soup. Reheat to serving temperature, if necessary, and serve hot using 1 cup per serving.

Nutritive values per serving:	CAL	CHO (gm)	PRO (gm)	FAT (gm)	NA (mg)
	150	8	20	2	447

Food exchanges per serving: 3 lean meat, 1 vegetable
Low-sodium diets: Omit salt. Use fresh tomatoes or tomatoes canned without salt.

VEGETABLE CHOWDER

Yields 7 cups—7 servings

2 tablespoons margarine
½ cup chopped onions
¼ cup chopped carrots
¼ cup chopped fresh green peppers
1 cup diced fresh white potatoes
1 cup cream-style corn
1 teaspoon salt
¹⁄₁₆ teaspoon black pepper
3 cups water
4 ounces sliced fresh or frozen Brussels sprouts
⅓ cup instant dry milk
2 tablespoons flour
1 cup cold water

Melt margarine in the bottom of a saucepan. Add onions, carrots, and peppers and cook and stir over moderate heat until onions are soft but not browned.

Add potatoes, corn, seasonings, and water to vegetables. Bring to a boil. Reduce heat and simmer 20 minutes. Add Brussels sprouts to soup. Cover and simmer 10 minutes.

Stir milk, flour, and cold water together until smooth. Add to soup and stir to mix. Simmer, stirring frequently, for 3 minutes. Remove from heat and serve hot, 1 cup per serving.

Nutritive values per serving:	CAL	CHO (gm)	PRO (gm)	FAT (gm)	NA (mg)
	100	12	3	5	450

Food exchanges per serving: 2 vegetable, 1 fat
Low-sodium diets: Omit salt. Use salt-free margarine.

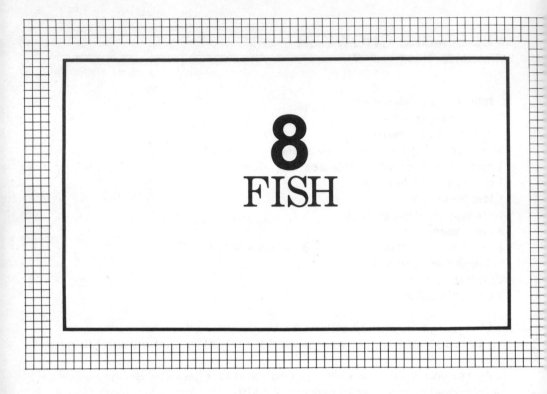

8
FISH

Fish is a wonderful food. It is low in calories and saturated fat, easy and quick to prepare, and comparatively inexpensive. With so many different kinds of fish available and so many different ways to prepare them, it is easy to have fish two or three times a week (as doctors and dietitians recommend) without repeating yourself very often. If you live along the coasts or in the Great Lakes area, you are probably used to serving a great deal of fish. If you live inland and aren't used to using all that much fish, you are going to be very pleasantly surprised as you try the various recipes and different kinds of fish available across the country.

Fish is available in the following forms:

- *Whole fish* are fish as they are caught. The fish needs to be scaled, eviscerated, and cut into portions, if necessary. The head and tail are generally removed although they may be left on some of the smaller fish.
- *Dressed fish* have had the scales and entrails removed. The head, tail, and fins are generally also removed although the head and tail may be left on smaller fish. These are called pan-dressed fish, such as trout or catfish. The fish may also be cut into fillets, steaks, or chunks.

- *Fillets* are ready to be cooked when they are purchased. They are the sides of fish cut from the backbone.
- *Steaks* are generally cut ⅝ to 1 inch thick and are cross sections cut from larger fish. The only bone in them is the cross section of the backbone. They are ready to be cooked when purchased.
- *Chunks* are cross section pieces of larger fish. The only bone that might be in them would be a cross section of the backbone, but most of the pieces are without bone. They are ready to be cooked when they are purchased.
- *Sticks and squares* are generally cut from frozen fish blocks. They are coated with a batter or breading. They are not recommended for a low-cholesterol diabetic diet unless you are sure the batter does not include whole eggs and the package includes nutritive information to help you determine the exchanges for them.
- *Fish portions* are generally individual pieces of fish that have been dipped in batter or breading and frozen so they can be cooked or reheated without further preparation. They, too, are not recommended for a low-cholesterol diabetic diet unless you are sure the batter does not contain whole eggs and the package includes nutritive information to help you determine the exchanges for them.
- *Canned fish* includes many varieties of fish. They are ready to be used as purchased. The ones packed in water are lower in calories than the ones packed in oil. The most readily available canned fish are salmon, tuna, mackerel, and sardines. Several species of fish are marketed as tuna and all of them are equally desirable.

When you are buying fresh fish, it should be really fresh. Fresh fish should have the following characteristics:

- *Flesh* should be firm and not separated from the bones.
- *Odor* should be fresh and mild. Fish with a strong odor is probably older since the fish odor becomes more apparent with age.
- *Eyes* should be bright and clear. The eyes become sunken as the fish becomes stale.
- *Gills* should be red and free of slime.
- *Skin* should be shiny with the color unfaded. Older fish lose their iridescence and the color is faded.
- *Fish steaks or fillets* should be firm and have a fresh-cut appearance. There should be no trace of brown or drying around the edges.

When you are buying frozen fish, the following points are important:

- *Flesh* should be frozen solid when purchased. There should not be any discoloration or freezer burn.
- *Odor* should not be apparent. Fish that is frozen properly should have little or no odor. A strong fish odor indicates poor quality.
- *Wrappings* should be of moisture- and vapor-retardant materials. There should be little or no space between the fish and the wrappings. Wrappings should not be torn, dirty, or discolored.

After fish are purchased, they must be stored correctly to avoid loss of quality and possible food spoilage or poisoning.

- *Fresh fish* should be placed in the refrigerator immediately after they are purchased. They should be stored in the refrigerator at 35–40° F. and should be used within 48 hours after they are purchased.
- *Frozen fish* should be placed in the freezer in their original wrappings and stored at zero degrees or below. Fish should always be dated so you can use the oldest fish first and not have to contend with freezer burn on some package that got shoved to the back of the freezer. It is important to thaw fish correctly. A 1-pound package of fish should thaw in the refrigerator in about 24 hours, or in 1–2 hours under cold running water. I thaw fish in the microwave, placing it at defrost for 5–10 minutes for a 1-pound package. Fish should never be defrosted at room temperature because of the danger of food spoilage or food poisoning. Frozen fillets or steaks may be cooked without thawing if you allow a little more cooking time, but if they are to be breaded or baked, they should always be thawed before they are prepared.

Fish is cooked to develop flavor, soften the small amount of connective tissue, and make it easier to digest. Fish cooked at too high a temperature or for too long will be tough and dry and the flavor will be poor.

Deep-fat-fried fish is a favorite with many people, but it isn't all that good on a low-cholesterol diabetic diet—you can't be sure exactly how much fat the fish has absorbed or what ingredients are in the batter. If you are eating in a restaurant, it is a good idea to order plain broiled or baked fish, and if it is served with a sauce ask them to serve the fish with the sauce on the side. If you can, you should ask what they have used to baste the fish; it might be an oil-based marinade, but then again it might be lemon butter, which you wouldn't want to eat.

I have tried to include recipes in this chapter to illustrate the various methods for preparing fish. If you have a favorite recipe you want to use that doesn't contain cholesterol, you can calculate the exchanges from the information in Chapter 2.

Some fish do contain some fat, although most of the different kinds of fish are very lean. Fish that are considered lean include the following: catfish, cod, flounder, haddock, halibut, lake perch, ocean perch, pike, red snapper, sole, swordfish, and whiting.

Some recipes for preparing fish are methods more than individual recipes. These include the following:

Broiled fish. This is a form of dry heat cooking but the heat is more direct and intense than when fish is baked. It is best to use steaks, fillets, or pan-dressed fish about 1 inch thick because the intense heat will dry out thinner fish. The fish should be thawed and patted dry with a paper towel and should be brushed with an oil-based marinade or sauce while it is being broiled. The directions for your own broiler should be followed; however, it is a general rule that fish should be broiled about 3–4 inches from the source of heat. Thicker cuts should be broiled further from the heat than thinner cuts. The length of time for broiling depends upon the thickness of the fish to be broiled and the distance from the heat. It generally takes about 10–15 minutes before the fish flakes easily when tested with a fork. Fish do not generally need to be turned while they are being broiled, but thicker pieces such as whole fish should be turned and brushed with more marinade when they are about half-cooked. Always serve broiled fish very hot.

Charcoal-broiled fish. Fish are good for this type of cooking because they cook so quickly. Pan-dressed fish, fillets, and steaks are all suitable for broiling. The fish should be thawed and patted dry before it is broiled; and because it flakes easily, it is a good idea to use a well-greased, long-handled, hinged wire grill for your fish. Thicker cuts of fish are best because they will dry out less than the thinner cuts, but all of them should be basted generously before and during the cooking period. Fish are generally cooked about 4 inches from moderately hot coals for 15–20 minutes depending upon the thickness of the fish. French or Italian style dressings which are based on oil are good for basting the fish. It is not a good idea to baste fish with a sauce high in sugar because it burns easily—but since we would never do that anyway we won't need to worry about that type of marinade. Marinades used for both types of broiling should be calculated when food exchanges for the fish are calculated.

Poached fish. Poaching means to cook in a simmering liquid. The fish should be placed in a single layer in a shallow, wide pan such as a large frying pan and barely covered with liquid. The liquid can be fish stock, lightly salted water, white wine and water, or water with various herbs in it. It is important not to let the water boil and not to overcook the fish. The fish should cook in a simmering liquid, in a covered pan, about 10–15 minutes or until the fish flakes easily when tested with a fork. It can then be served warm or cold with a sauce, in a salad, or used for a casserole.

Steamed fish. Steamed fish is generally cooked with steam from hot water although some people like to add herbs to the water. It is a good way to cook fish to retain its natural flavor and juices. A steamer is best, but any deep pan with a tight cover may be used if you have a rack that fits in the pan. The rack is to keep the fish out of the water. The fish is placed on a rack over rapidly boiling water and allowed to steam for 10–15 minutes or until the fish flakes easily when tested with a fork. Steamed fish is generally served the same way as poached fish.

Fish cooked in foil. Individual fish portions may be baked in the oven or prepared on an outside grill in foil. Put a single portion of fish in a foil packet along with some sauce or margarine and thinly sliced vegetables. It cooks beautifully this way without getting any pans dirty and tastes delicious when it is finished. It takes longer on the grill than in the oven but either method is satisfactory. The fish should be cooked until it flakes easily when tested with a fork.

Of course, all of the above methods yield fish that should be calculated using 1 ounce of the cooked fish as 1 lean meat exchange plus whatever sauce you use on the fish.

The sauces served with fish can be murder. I generally ask for the sauce on the side when ordering fish. If I can see that it is based on sour cream or is high in egg yolks or some other forbidden ingredient, I ask for lemon juice—or if all else fails, I ask for just plain vinegar. You would be surprised at the difference between those sauces and herb-flavored vinegar or lemon juice when you are calculating the exchanges for a fish recipe.

I first discovered the advantages of vinegar with fish when I was eating fish and chips in Great Britain. When I came home, I tried it again and liked it as well as I did over there. I guess I had thought that maybe it was the atmosphere over there which made me like it; however, it worked just as well here, so I experimented with different types of vinegar and discovered I could make my own herb vinegar very easily. I steep about a tablespoon of herbs (fresh if possible) in a cup of vinegar for a few days or until it is as strong as I like it. Then I strain off the herbs, put my vinegar in a cruet, and keep it for the next time we have fish. I even like to use the pickle juice from Mrs. Riley's Pickles (see index) on fish.

BAKED FISH STEAK

Yields 1 pound—4 servings

1 pound halibut or salmon steak cut ⅝–1 inch thick
⅓ cup Spicy Tomato Dressing (see index)

Defrost fish if necessary. Pat dry with paper towels. Line a small pan with aluminum foil. Grease the foil with margarine and place the steak on the pan. The steak can be cut into 4 equal portions at this time or after it is baked.

Brush steak generously with dressing using a pastry brush. Bake 25–35 minutes at 350° F. or until fish flakes easily when tested with a fork. Cut into 4 equal portions, if not already cut, and serve hot using 1 portion per serving.

Nutritive values per serving:

	CAL	CHO (gm)	PRO (gm)	FAT (gm)	NA (mg)
	146	2	24	4	112

Food exchanges per serving: 3 lean meat
Low-sodium diets: Use the low-sodium variation of the salad dressing.

BAKED FISH WITH MUSTARD SAUCE

Yields 6 fillets—6 servings

6 3-ounce fillets of codfish, haddock, perch, flounder, or whiting
Margarine
1 tablespoon lemon juice
1 tablespoon vegetable oil
1 teaspoon paprika
1 teaspoon salt
¼ cup all-purpose flour
2 tablespoons margarine
2 tablespoons instant dry milk
2 cups cool water
1 tablespoon chopped parsley
2 teaspoons salad mustard
Whisper of white pepper

Defrost fish if necessary. Pat dry with paper towels and place in a shallow baking pan lined with aluminum foil and greased with margarine.

In a small cup mix together lemon juice, oil, paprika, and ½ teaspoon of the salt. Using a pastry brush, brush the tops and sides of the fillets with the mixture. Bake at 350° F. for 30–40 minutes depending upon the thickness of the fillets, or until the fish flakes easily when tested with a fork.

While the fish is baking, in a small saucepan cook the flour, margarine, dry milk, and remaining ½ teaspoon salt. Stir over low heat until smooth. Add 2 cups water to flour mixture and cook and stir until smooth and thickened.

Add remaining seasonings to sauce and stir to mix well. Serve ⅓ cup hot sauce over 1 hot fish fillet per serving.

Nutritive values per serving using codfish:	CAL	CHO (gm)	PRO (gm)	FAT (gm)	NA (mg)
	150	6	16	7	478

Food exchanges per serving: 2 lean meat, ½ milk
Low-sodium diets: Omit salt. Use salt-free margarine.

CODFISH WITH MUSHROOM SAUCE

Yields 4 fillets—4 servings

1 4-ounce can mushroom stems and pieces
2 tablespoons margarine
2 tablespoons all-purpose flour
¼ teaspoon salt
Whisper of white pepper
1 cup fat-free chicken broth
4 4-ounce codfish fillets

Drain mushrooms well. Discard juice and chop mushrooms into smaller pieces, if necessary. Place in small saucepan. Add margarine, flour, and seasonings to mushrooms and cook and stir over moderate heat until lightly browned. Add broth to mushrooms. Cook and stir over moderate heat until smooth and thickened.

Thaw fish if necessary. Pat dry with a paper towel and place in a 1½-quart casserole. Cover with the hot sauce, using a fork to ease the sauce around the fish. Bake uncovered at 350° F. for 30–35 minutes or until the fish flakes easily when tested with a fork. Serve 1 fillet and a little of the sauce per serving.

Nutritive values per serving:

CAL	CHO (gm)	PRO (gm)	FAT (gm)	NA (mg)
158	5	21	6	636

Food exchanges per serving: 1 vegetable, 3 lean meat
Low-sodium diets: Omit salt. Use salt-free margarine, low-sodium broth, and fresh mushrooms.

FISH CREOLE

Yields 4 fillets—4 servings

4 4-ounce fillets of codfish, haddock, perch, flounder, or whiting
2 tablespoons vegetable oil
¼ cup chopped fresh green peppers
¼ cup chopped onions
1 tablespoon all-purpose flour
1 cup chopped canned tomatoes and juice
½ teaspoon salt
½ teaspoon sugar
⅛ teaspoon ground cloves
Whisper of pepper

Defrost fish, if necessary. Pat dry with paper towels and place in a shallow 1-quart casserole.

Place oil in a small saucepan. Bring to a cooking temperature. Add peppers and onions and cook, stirring frequently, over moderate heat until onions are soft but not browned. Add flour to vegetables. Cook and stir until flour is absorbed by the vegetables.

Add tomatoes and seasonings to vegetables. Cook and stir over moderate heat for 2 minutes. Pour the hot sauce over the fish. Bake, uncovered, at 350° F. for 35–40 minutes or until the fish flakes easily when tested with a fork. Serve hot using 1 fillet and some of the sauce per serving.

Nutritive values per serving using codfish:	CAL	CHO (gm)	PRO (gm)	FAT (gm)	NA (mg)
	176	6	21	7	427

Food exchanges per serving: 1 vegetable, 3 lean meat
Low-sodium diets: Omit salt. Use low-sodium canned tomatoes or fresh tomatoes.

OVEN-FRIED FISH FILLETS

Yields 8 fillets—8 servings

3 tablespoons margarine at room temperature
½ cup dry bread crumbs
1 teaspoon paprika
¼ teaspoon garlic powder
½ teaspoon salt
2 tablespoons Parmesan cheese
8 4-ounce codfish fillets
½ cup skim milk

Line a 9″ × 13″ cake pan with aluminum foil. Grease the foil using part of the margarine. Set the remaining margarine aside for later use.

Place bread crumbs, seasonings, and Parmesan in a pie pan. Mix well to blend and set aside for later use.

Defrost fish if necessary. Pat dry with a paper towel. Place milk in an individual salad bowl. Dip fish fillets in milk and then in the bread crumb mixture. Place evenly on the foil in the pan.

Using all the remaining margarine, spread a small amount of the margarine on top of each of the fillets. Bake at 500° F. for 10–15 minutes or until lightly browned and firm. (The length of time will depend upon the thickness of the fillets.) Let stand 5 minutes and serve hot, using 1 fillet per serving.

Nutritive values per serving:	CAL	CHO (gm)	PRO (gm)	FAT (gm)	NA (mg)
	162	5	22	5	331

Food exchanges per serving: 1 vegetable, 3 lean meat
Low-sodium diets: Omit salt. Use salt-free margarine.

SHRIMP ETOUFFEE

Yields 3 cups—3 servings

This is another Cajun recipe I developed, with the help of Della Andreassen, R.D., from Lafayette, Louisiana, for an article about Cajun cooking for DITN (Diabetes in the News).

1 tablespoon vegetable oil
¾ cup chopped onions
½ cup chopped fresh green peppers
½ cup chopped celery
½ cup tomato sauce
¼ cup water
2 teaspoons cornstarch
⅛–¼ teaspoon cayenne pepper
¼ teaspoon salt
8 ounces cooked, cleaned shrimp
¼ cup chopped fresh green onion tops

Preheat ½-quart saucepan over medium heat for 1 minute. Swirl oil in bottom of pan. Add onions, green peppers, and celery and cook, stirring frequently, over medium heat until onions are soft but not browned.

In a separate bowl combine tomato sauce, water, cornstarch, cayenne pepper, and salt and stir until smooth. Add tomato sauce mixture to vegetables and cook and stir until sauce is clear. Add shrimp and heat to serving temperature. Stir chopped onion tops into mixture and serve hot using 1 cup per serving. *Note:* This is good over rice, but rice is not included in the nutritive analysis.

Nutritive values per serving:	CAL	CHO (gm)	PRO (gm)	FAT (gm)	NA (mg)
	204	8	17	6	1,932

Food exchanges per serving: 2 lean meat, ½ bread
Low-sodium diets: This recipe is not suitable.

SALMON PATTIES WITH CREAMED PEAS

Yield 6 patties—6 servings

1 1-pound can red salmon
2 large egg whites
1 tablespoon finely chopped onions
¼ teaspoon salt
Whisper of pepper
1 cup crushed white soda crackers or saltines
1 cup fat-free chicken broth
1 tablespoon cornstarch
1 tablespoon margarine
1½ cups drained canned peas

Drain salmon and place the juice in a mixing bowl. Remove bones and dark skin from the salmon and set aside. Add egg whites, onions, salt, and pepper to salmon juice and mix together with a fork.

Crush the crackers with your hands. Do not use cracker crumbs. Add to the egg white mixture along with the salmon. Mix well with a fork to blend. (The cracker pieces and small chunks of salmon should still be visible.) Shape into patties about ¾ inch thick using about ⅓ cup of the mixture per patty. Place patties on a small cookie sheet that has been greased with margarine. Bake at 350° F. for 35–40 minutes or until firm and lightly browned.

Stir broth and cornstarch together until smooth. Cook and stir over moderate heat in a small saucepan until thickened and smooth. Continue to cook and stir for another minute. Add margarine and peas to sauce and mix lightly. Reheat to serving temperature. Serve 1 patty with ⅙ of the sauce (about ⅓ cup) per serving.

Nutritive values per serving:

CAL	CHO (gm)	PRO (gm)	FAT (gm)	NA (mg)
204	14	19	10	866

Food exchanges per serving: 1 bread, 2 lean meat
Low-sodium diets: Omit salt. Use salt-free margarine, low-sodium crackers, and fresh or frozen peas. Discard salmon juice and substitute an equal amount of water.

TUNA FISH, MUSHROOMS, AND CELERY

Yield 4 cups—6 servings

If you have wondered why I use mushrooms and celery so often, it is not only because we like them but also because they add bulk and flavor to a recipe without adding much carbohydrate or many calories.

2 6½-ounce cans of chunk-style tuna fish packed in water
3 tablespoons margarine
1 cup thinly sliced celery
1 4-ounce can mushroom stems and pieces, drained
3 tablespoons all-purpose flour
2 cups water at room temperature
½ cup instant dry milk
½ teaspoon salt
Whisper of white pepper

Drain tuna well. Discard liquid and set tuna fish aside for later use.

Place margarine in a 1½ quart saucepan. Melt over moderate heat. Add celery and mushrooms and cook, stirring occasionally, over moderate heat until celery is limp. Add flour to vegetables and cook and stir until flour is absorbed.

With a fork, mix water, dry milk, salt, and pepper to blend. Add to vegetables and cook and stir over moderate heat until smooth and thickened. Add tuna fish. Mix very lightly and serve hot using ¾ cup per serving.

Nutritive values per serving:	CAL	CHO (gm)	PRO (gm)	FAT (gm)	NA (mg)
	179	6	20	8	381

Food exchanges per serving: ½ milk, 2 lean meat
Low-sodium diets: Omit salt. Use salt-free margarine.

TARTAR SAUCE

Yields 1¼ cups—10 servings

1 cup Kay's Cooked Dressing (see index)
2 tablespoons finely chopped Mrs. Riley's Pickles (see index)
1 tablespoon finely chopped onions
1 tablespoon chopped pimientos
1 tablespoon chopped parsley

Mix all ingredients well to blend. Refrigerate until served, using 2 table-spoons per serving.

Nutritive values per serving:

CAL	CHO (gm)	PRO (gm)	FAT (gm)	NA (mg)
23	2	negl.	1	45

Food exchanges per serving: 2 tablespoons may be considered free.
Low-sodium diets: Use low-sodium variation of salad dressing.

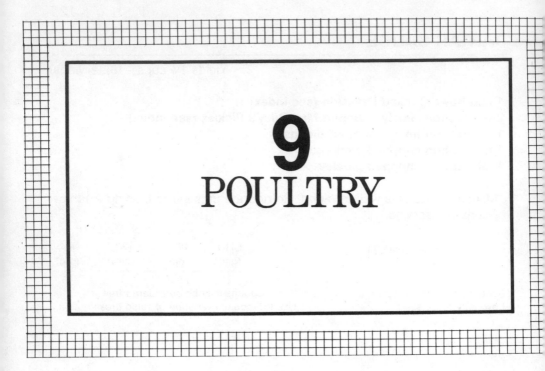

9
POULTRY

Chicken and turkey are both important in the low-cholesterol diabetic diet because they are low in calories, easily available, and comparatively inexpensive. It is also relatively simple to remove the skin and fat from them before they are cooked. Goose is a little too fat and I never use it, but I depend upon chicken and turkey for many of our meals.

Chicken and turkey are interchangeable in many recipes and especially so when you are using cubed or diced, raw or cooked chicken or turkey with the fat and skin removed. When they are used interchangeably in recipes the nutritive values are based upon the first one listed. However, the food exchanges do not vary when one or the other is used.

Giblets should never be used on a low-cholesterol diet. If you don't have someone in your family who can use them, save them for a friend or neighbor who doesn't have to worry about cholesterol or give them to your cat or dog—they'll probably love them.

All poultry is perishable and you should be careful when you are buying or storing it. It is a good idea to always observe the following precautions:

1. Buy frozen or chilled poultry only from freezers or refrigerated cases.
2. Inspect the wrappers to be sure they are not torn or damaged.

126

3. Keep fresh poultry in the coldest part of your refrigerator; use it within two days after it is purchased or freeze it for later use.

Chicken or turkey parts may be purchased and they are often a better buy than the whole chicken or turkey. Turkey breast makes a very good roast and has less waste than the whole turkey. One ounce of the cooked turkey roast, without any skin, is of course 1 lean meat exchange. You can also buy turkey legs or thighs. I cook them all afternoon in the crockpot and then use the meat for turkey sandwiches, à la king, casseroles, or salads if I have any left after dinner. Turkey frankfurters are available and they are better for a low-cholesterol diet than regular frankfurters—but they still aren't really all that good for you because they do have fat in them. Turkey ham is lean and I buy that occasionally because it is generally lower in fat than regular ham.

I haven't included directions for roasting a turkey because most of the turkeys you buy include that information on the wrapper. However, I want to caution you not to cook the dressing inside the chicken or turkey for a low-cholesterol diet. It picks up too much fat that way—saturated fat that is not acceptable on a low-cholesterol diet. I know it is good that way, and that is probably how your grandmother did it, but it is better to cook the dressing in a separate pan where you can control the amount and kind of fat in the dressing. If you cook dressing inside the chicken or turkey, give it to someone who doesn't need to worry about cholesterol—and prepare yours in a separate pan.

I remove the skin from a chicken before I roast it, but I don't when I roast a turkey. It is simple to serve a slice of the turkey breast with very little of the fat from the skin on it, but it isn't all that easy on the smaller chicken.

In my role as dietary consultant, every year I discuss the sanitation measures to be taken when preparing poultry with the dietary staff at the Lutheran Home in Strawberry Point, Iowa. This year one of the ladies told me she thought she could give the lecture because she had heard it so many times—so I asked each of them to give the group a point that they remembered. I was pleased to find that they were all well aware of the precautions we should take when preparing poultry. The points we covered included the following:

1. *Be careful that everything is scrubbed* including table tops, chopping boards, knives, pans, and anything which might touch the poultry—both before and after you work with raw poultry.

2. *Do not defrost poultry at room temperature.* It should be defrosted in the refrigerator even if it does take several days for a large turkey. If you

don't have refrigerator space sufficient to keep a large turkey in the refrigerator for that long, it can be defrosted, still in its plastic bag, in the sink in cold running water. This will take several hours but can be done the day before you want to cook the turkey.

3. *Do not stuff chicken or turkey the night before it is to be cooked,* or stuff it and cook it partially one day and finish cooking it the next day. Prestuffing gives bacteria a chance to multiply and could cause food poisoning.

4. *As soon as possible after dinner, refrigerate leftover chicken or turkey, dressing, and gravy in a shallow pan.* Food stored in a deep pan takes too long to cool to the correct temperature and bacteria can develop while it is chilling. Don't let chicken or turkey, dressing, or gravy stay on the table at room temperature for nibbling after dinner. Refrigerate everything as soon as possible and if anyone wants a snack, let him go to the refrigerator for it, or set it out for guests to help themselves later.

5. *Leftover chicken or turkey should be frozen if it is not to be used within the next couple of days.* Divide it into serving-size portions and freeze it for future use. It is a big help when you have unexpected company or want to make yourself a different entrée than you are serving to others in the family. I don't like to carry a chicken or turkey sandwich for lunch because of the danger of bacterial contamination, but if you freeze the sandwich and wrap it in foil it will be cold enough to be safe several hours later when you need it.

I hope you will enjoy the recipes in this chapter. Chicken and turkey are a very special treat in many parts of the world and you can make them a special treat in your home, also. If you have a recipe of your own that you want to use, calculate the nutritive values in the recipe using the information in Chapter 2, and then go on from there. Remember to remove the skin and fat before the chicken is cooked and don't use any butter, cream, eggs, or other no-nos in your recipe.

ROAST CHICKEN

Yield 18 ounces cooked chicken—6 servings

I like leftovers. They are so nice to have on hand and I especially like leftover roast chicken—it makes such good sandwiches, salads, or casse roles. It is almost impossible these days to get an old-fashioned roasting chicken, which is good because those heavier chickens have a very high percentage of the fat we are trying to avoid on a low-cholesterol diabetic diet. Look for the heavier broiler-fryers and you should be able to find one weighing 3½ pounds, big enough for roasting.

1 3½-pound broiler-fryer chicken

Wash chicken well. Remove all skin and visible fat with a sharp knife. (Give the giblets to your cat or cook for someone who isn't on a low-cholesterol diet.) Place the chicken on a rack in a small roaster, breast side down. Cover and roast at 325° F. for 1½–1¾ hours or until tender and lightly browned. Remove from the oven and let set 15 minutes before it is carved into portions. (*Note:* If you want to serve ¼ of a chicken, start out with a 2½-pound broiler-fryer and roast it about 1½ hours, cut it into 4 equal portions, and serve ¼ of the chicken per serving.) Serve 3 ounces of boneless cooked chicken per serving.

Nutritive values per serving:	CAL	CHO (gm)	PRO (gm)	FAT (gm)	NA (mg)
	112	negl.	20	3	156

Food exchanges per serving: 3 lean meat
Low-sodium diets: May be used as written.

OVEN-BROWNED CHICKEN

Yields 1 chicken—4 servings

This is the chicken that Chuck and our neighbor, Garrieth "Butch" Franks, prefer, and they especially like it with rice cooked in chicken broth.

1 2½-pound broiler-fryer chicken
¾ cup dry bread crumbs
1 teaspoon salt
2 teaspoons paprika
¹⁄₁₆ teaspoon black pepper
½ teaspoon rubbed sage or thyme
1 large egg white
½ cup water
1 tablespoon margarine
1 tablespoon vegetable oil

Wash chicken well. Remove skin and all visible fat with a sharp knife and cut into serving-size pieces. You should have 2 breast halves, 2 thighs, and 2 legs. (Freeze the neck, wings, and back to use later to make chicken broth.)

Mix bread crumbs and seasonings well and place in a pie pan. (You won't need but about half of this amount, but you need a certain amount in order to be able to dredge the chicken in it successfully. Discard the remainder. Nutritive values are calculated using ½ of the bread crumb mixture.)

Mix egg white and water well and put into an individual salad bowl. Spread a small rimmed cookie sheet with aluminum foil and spread the margarine on the aluminum foil. Dip each piece of chicken in the egg white mixture and then dredge it in the bread crumb mixture and place on the aluminum foil.

Dribble ½ teaspoon oil on the top of each piece of chicken. Bake at 350° F. for 30 minutes. Remove the chicken from the oven. Turn it over and continue to bake for another 30 minutes. Serve hot or cold using 1 breast half or 1 leg and 1 thigh per serving.

Nutritive values per serving:	CAL	CHO (gm)	PRO (gm)	FAT (gm)	NA (mg)
	215	7	23	10	435

Food exchanges per serving: 3 lean meat, ½ bread
Low-sodium diets: Omit salt. Use salt-free margarine.

POACHED CHICKEN

Yields 1 chicken—4 servings

The poaching liquid can be changed to suit your favorite seasonings without changing the nutritive values, as long as it is based on chicken broth and no fat is added.

1 2½-pound broiler-fryer chicken
1 cup fat-free chicken broth
¼ teaspoon thyme or sage
¼ teaspoon salt
1 teaspoon chopped parsley
2 tablespoons orange juice
¼ cup dry white wine

Wash chicken well; remove skin and all visible fat with a sharp knife and cut into 4 equal portions. Place chicken in a shallow casserole. Discard the giblets, or give them to someone who isn't worried about cholesterol.

Mix together remaining ingredients and pour over chicken. Cover tightly with aluminum foil and bake at 325° F. for about 1 hour or until the chicken is tender. Remove from oven and serve ¼ chicken per serving. (Discard the poaching liquid. It is too highly spiced to be good for soup and it isn't thick enough or flavorful enough for a sauce on the chicken.)

Nutritive values per serving:	CAL	CHO (gm)	PRO (gm)	FAT (gm)	NA (mg)
	146	2	21	3	432

Food exchanges per serving: 3 lean meat
Low-sodium diets: Omit salt. Use salt-free chicken broth.

EMPEROR CHICKEN BREASTS

Yields 4 chicken breast halves with sauce—4 servings

This recipe comes from the multitalented "Chef Dave."

¼ teaspoon **Chinese Five Spice seasoning (found in the ethnic food section of most stores)**
Soy sauce
4 4-ounce boneless, skinless chicken breast halves
1 tablespoon stick margarine
¼ **cup cornstarch**
¼ **cup all-purpose flour**
2½ **cups fat-free chicken broth**
¼ **cup soy sauce**
2 tablespoons cornstarch
2 tablespoons brown sugar
3 finely chopped garlic cloves
1 tablespoon peanut oil
1 teaspoon finely minced fresh ginger
½ **cup chopped onions**
½ **cup chopped fresh green peppers**
½ **cup chopped celery**
½ **cup coarsely grated carrots**
1 8-ounce can sliced bamboo shoots
1 cup coarsely chopped Chinese cabbage or bok choy
1 to 2 teaspoons Weight Watchers dry sugar substitute

Combine Chinese Five Spice seasoning and soy sauce in a shallow baking pan. Wash chicken, drain well, and marinate overnight in soy sauce mixture. Drain well. Use ¼ of the margarine to grease a 9-inch-square hard-surface, nonstick pan. Set aside.

Blend ¼ cup cornstarch and flour in a shallow dish. Dredge chicken in flour mixture. Shake off any excess flour mixture and place chicken in the greased pan. Divide remaining margarine into 4 equal portions and put 1 portion on top of each breast half. Bake, uncovered, at 375° F. for 30–40 minutes, or until browned.

While chicken is baking, combine chicken broth, ¼ cup soy sauce, 2 tablespoons cornstarch, brown sugar, and garlic. Blend well and set aside.

Preheat a hard-surface, nonstick frying pan, add peanut oil and ginger and cook and stir over medium heat until you can smell the ginger. Add onions, green peppers, celery, carrots, bamboo shoots, and Chinese cabbage or bok choy. Cook and stir over medium heat about 5 minutes or until thickened and lightly browned. Mix lightly and pour over browned chicken.

Bake, uncovered, at 325° F. for 30 minutes or until chicken is lightly browned. Serve hot, using ½ breast topped with ¼ of chicken broth mixture and ¼ of vegetable mixture for each serving.

	CAL	CHO (gm)	PRO (gm)	FAT (gm)	NA (mg)
Nutritive values per serving:	285	17	30	8	2,024

Food exchanges per serving: 1 bread, 4 lean meat
Low-sodium diets: Omit salt and use salt-free broth.

CHICKEN OR TURKEY MUSHROOM CASSEROLE

Yields 3 cups—4 servings

1 4-ounce can mushroom stems and pieces
1 10¾-ounce can Campbell's Cream of Chicken soup
½ cup fat-free chicken broth
1 cup diced cooked chicken or turkey without skin or visible fat
½ cup long-grain rice
1 teaspoon chopped parsley

Combine mushrooms, soup, and broth in a small saucepan. Cook and stir over moderate heat until smooth and bubbling.

Add chicken, rice, and parsley to hot soup mixture. Stir to mix well and place in a 1½-quart casserole. Cover tightly and bake at 325° F. for 40 minutes or until rice is tender. Serve ¾ cup hot casserole per serving.

	CAL	CHO (gm)	PRO (gm)	FAT (gm)	NA (mg)
Nutritive values per serving:	224	25	15	7	781

Food exchanges per serving: 1 bread, 1 milk, 1 lean meat, 1 fat
Low-sodium diets: Use Campbell's low-sodium Cream of Chicken Soup and low-sodium broth.

MICROWAVE CHICKEN

Yields 1 chicken—4 servings

This recipe from Dr. Crockett is simple to prepare but it has an intriguing flavor. It can also be baked in a conventional oven, if you prefer.

1 2½-pound broiler-fryer chicken
½ teaspoon salt
¼ teaspoon ground sage
¾ cup orange juice
½ cup dry white wine

Wash chicken well. Remove all skin and visible fat with a sharp knife and cut into pieces. You should have 2 breast halves, 2 thighs, 2 wings, 2 legs, and the back. Freeze the wings, back, and neck for use for making broth later. Discard the giblets or give them to someone who isn't worried about cholesterol. Place the remaining pieces in an 8- or 9-inch dish suitable for use in the microwave.

Sprinkle salt and sage evenly over the chicken. Pour orange juice and wine over chicken pieces. Cover with plastic wrap or wax paper and cook on high for 5 minutes. Reduce heat to simmer and cook for 15–20 minutes or until tender. Serve hot with a little bit of the juice. Serve 1 breast half or 1 leg and 1 thigh per serving.

Note: If you prefer to use a conventional oven, cover the pan tightly with aluminum foil and bake at 325° F. for 45 minutes–1 hour or until the chicken is tender. If you prefer, you can remove the foil the last 15 minutes to allow the chicken to brown a little.

Nutritive values per serving:	CAL	CHO (gm)	PRO (gm)	FAT (gm)	NA (mg)
	185	8	22	3	325

Food exchanges per serving: 3 lean meat, ½ bread
Low-sodium diets: Omit salt.

JAMBALAYA

Yields 5 cups—5 servings

This is a recipe I developed with help from my friend Della Andreassen for an article for DITN (Diabetes in the News).

1 tablespoon vegetable oil
½ cup chopped onions
½ cup chopped fresh green peppers
½ cup chopped celery
1 16-ounce can tomatoes and juice
1 cup fat-free chicken broth
½ cup long-grain rice
½ teaspoon salt
⅛–¼ teaspoon cayenne pepper, depending upon preference
1 tablespoon chopped parsley
½ teaspoon thyme
1½ cups boneless, chopped, cooked chicken with fat and skin removed
½ cup chopped cooked ham with all visible fat removed

Preheat a 2-quart saucepan over medium heat for 1 minute. Swirl oil in bottom of pan. Add onions, green peppers, and celery. Cook, stirring frequently, over medium heat until onions are soft but not browned. Add tomatoes and juice, broth, rice, salt, cayenne pepper, parsley, and thyme. Cook, uncovered, over low heat, stirring frequently, for 20–25 minutes, or until rice is tender. If mixture gets too dry, add hot water, ¼ cup at a time. Add chicken and ham and continue to cook until meat is heated through. Serve hot, using 1 cup per serving.

Nutritive values per serving:	CAL	CHO (gm)	PRO (gm)	FAT (gm)	NA (mg)
	224	23	18	6	551

Food exchanges per serving: 1½ bread, 2 lean meat
Low-sodium diets: Omit salt. Use low-sodium canned tomatoes and broth.

CHICKEN AND BROCCOLI

Yields 2 cups—3 servings

This recipe is based on one from Judy Ballantine of Greensboro, North Carolina. Judy is my cousin Virginia Ballantine's daughter-in-law. Judy is a diabetic, also, and does such interesting things with vegetables, and with her life—she is a marvelous artist. We were all so proud of her when she took a trip to China with her husband, Dr. Larry Ballantine, in spite of the fact that she is a type I diabetic and had to manage her insulin, diet, and exercise to fit their schedule while they toured China.

1 tablespoon cornstarch
1 tablespoon sherry or fat-free chicken broth
2 tablespoons soy sauce
½ cup fat-free chicken broth
⅛ teaspoon ground ginger
⅛ teaspoon garlic powder
2 medium-size chicken breast halves without skin or visible fat
1 tablespoon vegetable oil
½ cup sliced onions
2 cups (6 ounces) frozen broccoli cuts
½ cup fat-free chicken broth

Combine first 6 ingredients and mix until smooth to form a marinade. Bone chicken breasts. Freeze bones for later use in broth and cut chicken into bite-size pieces. Place in marinade and refrigerate for 1–4 hours. Drain well, reserving marinade for later use.

Fry chicken in vegetable oil in heavy frying pan until clear and firm. Remove chicken from frying pan with a slotted spoon, leaving as much of the fat as possible still in the frying pan. Add onions and broccoli to the fat in the frying pan. Slice any larger pieces to about ½-inch thickness. Cook and stir about 1 minute or until broccoli is thawed.

Add broth to vegetables, mix lightly, cover, and simmer for 5 minutes or until the broccoli is crisp-tender. Add marinade and cook and stir over moderate heat until sauce is thickened and clear. Add chicken and reheat to serving temperature. Serve ⅔ cup per serving over hot rice.

Nutritive values per serving without rice:	CAL	CHO (gm)	PRO (gm)	FAT (gm)	NA (mg)
	194	9	20	8	1,212

Food exchanges per serving: ½ fruit, 3 lean meat

Low-sodium diets: Substitute ¼ cup lemon juice for the soy sauce and use ¼ teaspoon thyme instead of the ground ginger.

CHICKEN OR TURKEY À LA KING

Yields 4 cups—4 servings

1 4-ounce can mushroom stems and pieces
2 tablespoons vegetable oil
3 cups fat-free chicken broth
3 tablespoons cornstarch
¼ cup instant dry milk
⅛ teaspoon white pepper
2 cups cooked diced chicken or turkey with fat and skin removed
¼ cup chopped drained pimiento

Drain mushrooms well. Discard juice. Place oil in the bottom of a saucepan. Add the mushrooms and cook and stir over moderate heat until mushrooms are lightly browned.

Mix together broth, cornstarch, dry milk, and pepper until smooth. Add all at once to mushrooms and oil and stir, cooking over moderate heat until thickened. Continue to cook and stir another 2 minutes or until the starchy taste is gone.

Add chicken and pimiento to sauce. Mix lightly. Reheat to serving temperature and serve 1 cup per serving.

Nutritive values per serving:	CAL	CHO (gm)	PRO (gm)	FAT (gm)	NA (mg)
	235	9	23	12	890

Food exchanges per serving: ½ bread, 3 lean meat

Low-sodium diets: Use low-sodium chicken broth.

TOMATO CHICKEN SAUCE FOR SPAGHETTI

Yields 3 cups—6 servings

6 ounces raw boneless chicken without skin or visible fat
2 tablespoons vegetable oil
½ cup chopped onions
½ cup chopped fresh green peppers
½ cup chopped celery
2 cups canned tomato sauce
¼ teaspoon Italian seasoning
¼ teaspoon salt
¼ teaspoon leaf oregano
¼ teaspoon basil
½ teaspoon paprika
Whisper of white pepper

Cut chicken in ½-inch cubes and set aside for later use.

Place oil in the bottom of a saucepan. Heat over moderate heat for 1 minute. Add onions, peppers, celery, and chicken and cook and stir about 5 minutes or until chicken is white and firm, and vegetables are softened but not browned.

Add remaining ingredients to vegetables and chicken and cook, stirring almost constantly, for 5 minutes. Serve hot, ½ cup per serving, over hot spaghetti or hot, thin, homemade noodles.

Nutritive values per serving:	CAL	CHO (gm)	PRO (gm)	FAT (gm)	NA (mg)
	203	10	10	14	350

Food exchanges per serving without spaghetti or noodles: 1 lean meat, 2 vegetables, 2 fat

Low-sodium diets: Omit salt. Use tomato sauce canned without salt.

CHICKEN OR TURKEY CHOP SUEY

Yields about 6 cups—6 servings

2 tablespoons cornstarch
1⅓ cups cold fat-free chicken broth
2 tablespoons soy sauce
1 teaspoon sugar
1 cup celery cut into ½-inch pieces
½ cup sliced onions
1 4-ounce can mushroom stems and pieces with juice
2 cups (16-ounce can) drained bean sprouts
2 cups diced, cooked chicken or turkey with skin and fat removed

Place cornstarch, broth, soy sauce, and sugar in saucepan and mix until smooth. Add celery, onions, and mushrooms to chicken broth mixture. Bring to a boil. Reduce heat and simmer, stirring frequently, for 20 minutes. Add bean sprouts to vegetables and simmer another 5 minutes, stirring frequently.

Add chicken to vegetables. Reheat to serving temperature, if necessary, and serve over hot rice, using ⅙ of the recipe (about 1 cup) per serving.

Nutritive values per serving without rice:

CAL	CHO (gm)	PRO (gm)	FAT (gm)	NA (mg)
120	8	16	3	783

Food exchanges per serving: 2 lean meat, ½ bread

Low-sodium diets: This recipe is not suitable since the sauce is high in sodium because of the soy sauce— and it wouldn't be chop suey without the soy sauce.

CHICKEN AND BEAN SPROUTS WITH MUSHROOMS

Yields 3 cups—4 servings

1 4-ounce can mushroom pieces
Fat-free chicken broth as necessary
3 tablespoons soy sauce
1 teaspoon sugar
1½ tablespoons cornstarch
1 tablespoon sherry
2 tablespoons mushroom juice/chicken broth mixture
2 large chicken breast halves without skin or visible fat
2 tablespoons vegetable oil
1 16-ounce can bean sprouts

Drain mushrooms. Set drained mushrooms aside. Place the mushroom juice in a 1 cup measure and add enough broth to total 1 cup liquid. Set aside.

Mix together soy sauce, sugar, cornstarch, sherry, and 2 tablespoons of broth mixture in a small bowl until smooth, and set aside. Bone chicken breasts. You should have about 8 ounces chicken. Discard bones and cut chicken into ¾-inch cubes. Place chicken into the soy sauce mixture and let marinate for 10 minutes. Drain well, reserving the marinade for later.

Place oil in a heavy frying pan and heat over moderate heat until oil has a haze over it. Add the chicken to the hot oil and fry over moderate heat until chicken is firm and white, stirring frequently. Push chicken to the side of the frying pan. Add mushrooms and cook and stir until mushrooms are hot but not browned. Add chicken and mix lightly. Add remainder of marinade and chicken broth mixture and cook and stir over moderate heat until the sauce is thickened and clear.

Drain bean sprouts well and stir into chicken and sauce. Cook and stir until hot and the sprouts are covered with sauce. Serve hot over rice, using ¾ cup per serving.

Nutritive values per serving without rice:	CAL	CHO (gm)	PRO (gm)	FAT (gm)	NA (mg)
	210	9	20	10	1,374

Food exchanges per serving: 2 vegetable, 2 lean meat, 1 fat
Low-sodium diets: This recipe is not suitable since the sauce is high in sodium from the soy sauce, and the sauce would not be good without soy sauce.

CHICKEN OR TURKEY LOAF

Yields 1 loaf—12 servings

This makes excellent sandwiches, hot or cold.

2 pounds ground raw chicken or turkey
1 cup dry bread crumbs
2 large egg whites
2 chicken bouillon cubes dissolved in ½ cup water
1 tablespoon Worcestershire sauce or ½ teaspoon rubbed sage or thyme
1 tablespoon chopped parsley
¹/₁₆ teaspoon white pepper
½ cup finely chopped onions

It is best to grind the meat yourself since the ground chicken and turkey you buy generally has the skin and some fat in it. If your market will grind it for you without skin or fat you are in luck; but if not, figure that you will need about 3 pounds raw chicken or turkey for each pound of ground meat. Remove all skin and visible fat with a sharp knife. Bone the chicken or turkey, and then grind it in a meat grinder or chop it in a food processor. (Freeze the bones, wings, and neck to use to make broth later.) Refrigerate until needed. The ground poultry can also be used to make chicken or turkey patties.

Place remaining ingredients in mixing bowl. Mix well. Add chicken and mix lightly but thoroughly. Form into a loaf and place in a 9″ × 5″ × 3″ loaf pan that has been greased with margarine. Bake at 325° F. about 1½ hours or until firm and lightly browned. Remove from oven and let set for 15 minutes. Slice into 12 equal slices and serve 1 slice per serving.

Nutritive values per serving:	CAL	CHO (gm)	PRO (gm)	FAT (gm)	NA (mg)
	169	7	16	3	326

Food exchanges per serving: 2 lean meat, ½ bread
Low-sodium diets: Use ½ cup strong low-sodium fat-free chicken broth instead of the bouillon cubes and water. Use sage or thyme instead of Worcestershire sauce.

CHICKEN OR TURKEY SANDWICH SPREAD

Yields 1 cup—4 servings

This is a favorite of my neighbor Jan Franks. Beef may be substituted for the chicken with no change in the food exchanges, and that is the way she likes it best. This spread is also good for appetizers, and 1 tablespoon (about 3 appetizers) may be eaten without counting the spread.

1 cup diced, cooked chicken or turkey without skin or visible fat
3 tablespoons Kay's Cooked Dressing (see index)
2 tablespoons Mrs. Riley's Pickles, finely chopped (see index)

Chop chicken rather fine in a food processor or grind in a food grinder, using the coarse blade.

Add dressing and pickles to chicken and mix well. Refrigerate until served using ¼ cup per serving for a sandwich.

Nutritive values per serving:	CAL	CHO (gm)	PRO (gm)	FAT (gm)	NA (mg)
	77	2	11	2	76

Food exchanges per serving: 2 lean meat
Low-sodium diets: Use low-sodium variation of the salad dressing.

BREAD DRESSING

Yields 8-inch square pan—12 servings

This costs a lot in bread exchanges but I included it because it illustrates how to adapt bread dressing to a low-cholesterol diet. I like it well enough to consider it worth the bread exchanges it costs me.

2 tablespoons vegetable oil
¾ cup finely chopped celery
½ cup finely chopped onions
2 cups fat-free chicken or beef broth
¾ teaspoon ground sage or thyme
¹⁄₁₆ teaspoon black pepper
12 slices day-old white bread
2 egg whites

Place oil in the bottom of a saucepan. Add celery and onions and cook over moderate heat for 5 minutes, stirring frequently. Remove from heat. Add broth and seasonings to vegetables. Mix well and cool to lukewarm, if necessary.

Cut bread into cubes. It is a good idea to leave the bread spread out on a tray overnight before it is used—the bread won't absorb enough liquid to give it a good flavor if it isn't somewhat dry. Place cubes in a large mixing bowl.

Add egg whites to lukewarm vegetables and broth. Mix well and pour over bread cubes. Toss lightly but thoroughly. Spread evenly in an 8-inch square cake pan or 1-quart shallow casserole that has been well greased with margarine. Bake at 375° F. for 45 minutes. Cut 3 × 4 into 12 equal servings, allowing 1 square per serving.

Nutritive values per serving:	CAL	CHO (gm)	PRO (gm)	FAT (gm)	NA (mg)
	104	15	3	3	240

Food exchanges per serving: 1 bread, 1 fat
Low-sodium diets: Use salt-free broth.

CHICKEN OR TURKEY GRAVY

Yields 2 cups—8 servings

2¼ cups fat-free chicken or turkey drippings or broth
2 tablespoons cornstarch
⅛ teaspoon rubbed sage or thyme
1½ teaspoons margarine
Whisper of white pepper

Combine all ingredients in a small saucepan and cook and stir over moderate heat, stirring constantly, until thickened and smooth. Continue to cook and stir for another 2 minutes over low heat until the starchy taste is gone. Serve hot using ¼ cup gravy per serving. (The flavor of the gravy will depend upon the flavor of the drippings or broth, so it is a good idea to use the most flavorful drippings or broth possible for this gravy.)

	CAL	CHO (gm)	PRO (gm)	FAT (gm)	NA (mg)
Nutritive values per serving:	15	2	negl.	1	279

Food exchanges per serving: 1 serving may be considered free.
Low-sodium diets: Use low-sodium drippings or broth.

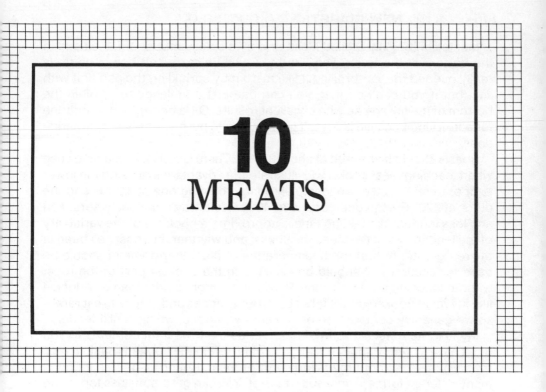

10
MEATS

Planning and preparing meat dishes is probably the hardest part of the low-cholesterol diabetic diet. Most of us are used to using a lot of plain roast meat, and this is still a good idea as long as we pick the leanest cuts and prepare them so that we remove as much of the remaining fat as possible.

Specific cuts with a lower fat content that are good for the low-cholesterol diabetic diet include the following:

- *Beef*—round, rump, sirloin, tenderloin, and dried beef
- *Pork*—loin, center cut roasts or chops, tenderloin, lean ham, center cut ham, and Canadian bacon
- *Veal*—round, rump, leg, sirloin, cutlets, and loin chops
- *Lamb*—sirloin, leg, cutlets, and sirloin chops

Baking, boiling, broiling, and roasting are all good methods for preparing meat because they help remove any remaining fat after all of the visible fat has been removed with a sharp knife. Baked or roasted meats should be placed on a rack so that the liquids will drip down in the bottom of the pan and the meat won't be cooking in its own fat. If necessary, the meat can be basted with broth or a marinade. Drippings in the bottom can be chilled and used for gravy or soups after the fat is removed.

Meats can be pan-broiled if salt or only a small amount of fat is used in the bottom of the frying pan—and you will be surprised how little fat is really needed for pan-broiling. I like to do it by sprinkling the pan first with salt; but if you can't do that, you can use just a tablespoon of oil in the bottom of the frying pan with excellent results. Oil is better than margarine for pan-frying because it doesn't get brown and burn as easily as margarine does.

Roasts should be cooked at about 325° F. There is a classic example I use when teaching meat cookery to illustrate the advantages of using the lower temperature: We take two identical roasts, roasting one at 325° F. and the other at 400° F.—the one cooked at 400° F. is always obviously shrunken and less tender. All roasting time is approximate because of the variability of the tenderness of the meat, thickness, and whether the roast has been in the refrigerator or is at room temperature. A meat thermometer should be used for accuracy. It should be inserted in the thickest part of the roast without touching any fat or bone. Rare meat is more tender than well done. I like my meat cooked until it falls apart, but Frances and Chuck like it rare—so we generally compromise on medium well done, which is still tender.

My favorite roast is round of beef. It has the lowest fat content, so you don't have to worry about the amount of fat left in the cooked roast. In fact, round of beef is about my favorite cut of meat. Round of beef is found in many different forms in your supermarket. You can get a boneless top round roast, eye of round roast, and the less tender bottom round pot roast. You can find thick round steaks for broiling and thinner round steaks for grilling or pan-frying. There are thinly sliced minute steaks for sandwiches, and top round can be found which has been cut into cubes for stews or broiling on skewers. The less tender bottom round can be cut into cubes or ground for use in spaghetti sauce, stew, or chili. Bottom round is also the top choice ground for hamburgers.

I must admit that roast round of beef requires a little extra care to make it tender. Top round or eye of round are best for roasting. Roast it, uncovered, at 300° F. to about 130–140° F. internally for rare or medium rare. Don't overcook it. Well done round of beef will be tough unless you pot-roast it until it is falling apart (which is the way I really prefer it, but that's another recipe). It is better if it is soaked in a marinade for several hours or overnight in the refrigerator—or a commercial tenderizer can be used according to the directions on the package. (Never use tenderizer on hamburger; it makes it mushy.) Don't bother to include oil in your marinade. It doesn't help tenderize the meat and adds calories and fat exchanges. Wine, vinegar, and tomato juice contain natural acids which tenderize meat without the addition of many calories.

Flank steak, rump, round, or sirloin tip are best used for stews and casseroles. If you must use stew meat, remove all visible fat before it is cooked. All stew meat should be browned first in as little fat as possible, covered with liquid, and simmered until tender. It can then be drained and the broth refrigerated until it is cool and the fat has risen to the top. I'm sure you will be surprised at the amount of fat you will be able to skim off the broth before it is recombined with the meat again and the stew or casserole finished. This is a time-consuming task, so I generally do several pounds of meat at once and then freeze what I'm not going to use that day in portions for future use.

Recipes including ground beef should be prepared so that you get as much of the fat as possible out of the meat. Buy lean ground beef, ground round of beef or veal, or ground leg of lamb. I try to use recipes which allow the meat to be browned, drained, and rinsed with hot water before it is combined with other ingredients. Meat loaves aren't all that good for you if they contain much filler such as bread crumbs or oatmeal, because the fillers absorb the saturated fat from the meat while the loaf is cooking. This is too bad because meat loaves are handy to have for sandwiches— besides, I really like a good meat loaf, and you probably do, too! Because meat loaves tend to hold fat, it is a good idea to use only the leanest meat in them, or chicken or turkey, which also make a good meat loaf (see index). The best way to do it when you want to make a beef meat loaf is to buy round steak, have the butcher remove any visible fat, and then grind the meat for you. If you don't have a butcher who will do it for you, a food processor will do a good job. Most heavy-duty mixers have good grinders, or you can buy an electric or hand grinder to use. If you grind the meat yourself you can be sure that you have removed all possible visible fat before grinding.

Hamburgers are good and we all love them, but it isn't a good idea to buy them out because the fat content is generally very high. If you do have to buy them at a hamburger stand, take a paper napkin and blot the fat off of both sides of the hamburger before you eat it. When you cook them at home you can cook them whatever way is most popular with your family, using lean ground meat and whatever seasonings you like; however, it is best not to add bread crumbs or other fillers to the meat because they trap the fat which you are trying to get rid of. It will taste good but it will have more saturated fat than you really should be using. Hamburgers can be prepared according to one of the following methods:

- *Grilled.* Heat a grill until it is sizzling hot, rub lightly with oil or sprinkle with salt (if permissible), and brown the burgers on both sides.

Reduce the heat and cook them over medium heat 2–8 minutes on each side depending upon whether you like them rare or well done.

- *Pan-fried.* Heat a heavy frying pan until sizzling hot, rub lightly with oil or sprinkle with salt (if permissible), and brown the burgers on both sides. Reduce the heat and cook them over medium heat 2–8 minutes on each side depending upon whether you like them rare or well done.
- *Broiled.* Arrange hamburger patties on a cold broiler rack. Broil 3–4 inches from the heat, turning once, for about 4–6 minutes on each side depending upon how thick they are and how well done you like them to be.

It is a good idea to stick to the *good* grade of beef. *Choice* beef may be a little more tender, but that is because it has more marbling of fat and this is what you want to avoid. Check the grade of beef before you buy it, and if you are in doubt always check with the butcher or salesman behind the counter. If it is practical for you, it is a good idea to buy your meat at a locker where you can be sure you are getting the *good* grade of beef, and then instruct them to remove every bit of fat possible before the meat is ground. This is what we do in our small town and it is really best if it is also possible in your area.

Swine breeders have developed much leaner hogs in the last few years, so that pork is no longer as fat as it used to be and may be used occasionally on a low-cholesterol diabetic diet. However, it is still wise to use the leanest cuts, avoiding spareribs, pork sausage, and other cuts, such as the shoulder, with a higher fat content. The tenderloin is particularly good and is luscious when cut thick and broiled as they do at the Chaparral, our local restaurant here in Wadena. Fresh ham and center cut loin are also good for roasting after all the visible fat has been removed. Pork chops should be center cut and have all visible fat removed before cooking, and they should not be cooked with dressing or stuffing because the dressing or stuffing picks up too much fat while they are baking.

Ham can be very lean, and if you don't have to worry about salt restrictions can be a very good buy, particularly some of the low-fat hams. Most hams available are precooked so you only need to reheat them to an interior temperature of 130° F. This should take about 15–20 minutes per pound at 325° F. or you can do it in the microwave, according to directions with your microwave. The center cut of smoked ham is generally acceptable also if all of the visible fat is removed. It may be broiled or pan-broiled.

- *Broiled.* Remove all visible fat from a center cut of ham about 1 inch thick. Broil about 15 minutes for precooked ham and about 25 minutes for uncooked ham, turning it once while it is broiling.
- *Pan-Broiled.* Remove all visible fat from a center cut of ham about ¼–½ inch thick. Rub a frying pan with a little oil and cook over medium heat, turning at least once while it is frying. Cook about 6–8 minutes for precooked ham and about 12–16 minutes for uncooked ham.

Here in Iowa we have what they call Iowa Pork Chops. These are lean chops that weigh about 8–9 ounces each. One chop is far too much for our meat allowance, but I like to brown them, put them in a small roaster with a rack, and continue cooking them, covered, in the oven at 325° F. for about an hour or until they are tender. I cut off the amount of meat that I am allowed for that meal and save the rest for another meal. It tastes like luscious roast pork and is really very good. If they aren't available in your area, I'm sure your butcher would be happy to cut some for you from the center loin. Of course, I cut off all visible fat before preparing them, and they are really very lean when prepared that way.

Properly cooked lamb has a delicious, mild flavor and an appetizing aroma. It should be served hot or cold—never lukewarm. In the past, recipes generally specified well-done lamb; however, today the accepted procedure is to cook it to 165° F., which is slightly rare. This gives you a more flavorful and juicy roast. Lamb is good for a low-cholesterol diet because it is lower in fat than many of the beef cuts. The leg is the leanest part of the lamb and it can be cut into a leg of lamb roast or a sirloin roast. The sirloin may also be cut into chops or ground. Lamb patties, which are traditionally lean, are often wrapped in bacon. We can't do this but I find that if I add a little seasoning and broil the patty until it is medium well done, it will be moist and juicy. If you buy the whole leg of lamb you will find it is covered with a whitish, brittle fat that is called the fell. This should be removed before the roast is cooked because it tends to make the flavor of the meat strong, as well as adding additional fat that you don't need.

Veal has a delicate flavor when it is cooked properly. Good veal is light pink in color rather than red and has a small amount of very white fat. It is not suited for broiling because of the small amount of fat, but that small amount of fat makes it an excellent choice for a low-cholesterol diabetic diet. Veal cutlets are very lean and may be pan-broiled. They are often dipped in egg white and then cracker crumbs and deep fat fried. This method would be satisfactory except that it does add more fat exchanges. The veal cutlets may also be dipped in egg white and then crumbs and pan-broiled using a very little oil, which uses fewer fat exchanges and still tastes like a good veal cutlet. Veal is a good choice for stews and casseroles because of its low fat content—and roast leg of veal is an excellent entrée for a dinner or special occasion.

If you have a favorite meat recipe that isn't included in this book, you can calculate the nutritive values for it using the information in Chapter 2. Roast meats are calculated using nutritive values of 1 meat exchange per 1 ounce serving of meat. If gravy is used it will have to be figured separately. I have not included many roast recipes in this book—there are so many of them in other cookbooks. I have used the space for casseroles and other combination dishes. When we were first talking about this book, Sister Rosemary, who is a dietitian at Holy Cross Hospital in Chicago, told me that she hoped I'd use mostly casseroles and similar recipes because that is what most of her patients want. I have tried to illustrate different methods of preparation hoping that you could use them as a basis for your own recipes—but remember, if you add or subtract something, unless it is very, very low in food value like celery or mushrooms, you must recalculate the recipe to arrive at the correct exchanges for your diet pattern.

BROILED ROUND STEAK

Yields 21 to 24 ounces

Who says we can't have steak on a low-cholesterol diet? I think you will be surprised when you taste this broiled steak.

It is really a method more than an exact recipe. You can vary the marinade to suit yourself, which will change the flavor a little bit. The steak will be more tender if it is rare or, at the least, medium done. This method also will work for a round bone pot roast, although the round is better for a low-cholesterol diet.

2 pounds round of beef, 2 inches thick, with all visible fat removed
¼ cup vegetable oil
¼ cup red wine vinegar
¼ cup red wine
¼ to ½ teaspoon garlic powder
1 teaspoon leaf thyme
1 teaspoon leaf oregano
3 tablespoons chopped parsley
Salt and pepper as necessary

Place steak in a shallow dish. Mix together all remaining ingredients except salt and pepper to blend and pour over the round steak. Cover tightly and let it marinate at room temperature for about 2 hours, or overnight in the refrigerator. Remove meat from the marinade. Pat it dry with a paper towel and discard the marinade. Broil 3–4 minutes on each side about 4 inches from the heat for rare, or more as desired.

Season meat with salt and pepper and serve hot. It can be carved in thin slices across the grain or served in large pieces for each person to cut his own. Food exchanges will depend upon the size servings, with 1 ounce cooked meat counted as one lean meat exchange. Low-sodium diets should omit the salt.

TEXAS ROUND STEAK

Yields 6 steaks—6 servings

½ cup all-purpose flour
1 teaspoon salt
1½ teaspoons chili powder
1 pound 2 ounces round of beef about ½ inch thick (weighed after fat
   and bone are removed), cut into 6 3-ounce steaks
2 tablespoons vegetable oil
½ cup chopped fresh green peppers
½ cup chopped onions
1 cup fat-free beef broth
½ cup tomato sauce
½ cup tomato juice
1 teaspoon chili powder
¼ teaspoon garlic powder
¼ teaspoon ground cumin

Blend flour, salt, and chili powder well and place in a pie pan. Dredge meat in the flour mixture. You should use about half of the mixture. (You can discard the rest; however, it is necessary to have this amount to make dredging practical.)

Place oil in a heavy frying pan and heat to frying temperature over moderate heat. Add meat and brown on both sides. Transfer steaks to a 1½-quart casserole.

Fry peppers and onions over moderate heat in the pan in which the meat was browned, stirring frequently. Remove vegetables with a slotted spoon and spread over the meat. Pour out any remaining fat. Add beef broth to frying pan and cook and stir over moderate heat to absorb any brown particles remaining in the pan.

Add remaining ingredients to broth. Mix well and pour over meat. Stir the meat and vegetables lightly with a fork to distribute the broth and vegetables. Cover tightly and bake at 325° F. for about 1–1½ hours or until the meat is tender. Serve 1 piece of steak with some of the sauce per serving.

Nutritive values per serving:	CAL	CHO (gm)	PRO (gm)	FAT (gm)	NA (mg)
	213	9	20	11	460

Food exchanges per serving: ½ fruit, 3 lean meat
Low-sodium diets: Omit salt. Use low-sodium broth, tomato sauce, and tomato juice.

BEEF WITH GREEN BEANS

Yields 3 cups—4 servings

I find this easier to prepare in an electric frying pan. I'm not sure why but I always prepare it that way.

8 ounces round of beef with all visible fat removed before it is weighed
2 tablespoons soy sauce
1 tablespoon cornstarch
½ teaspoon salt
1 tablespoon sherry or beef broth
1 tablespoon vegetable oil
¼ cup water
1 pound frozen green beans cut into 1-inch lengths

Cut beef into pieces about ⅛–¼ inch thick and about 1 inch long. (This is easier if the meat is slightly frozen.) Refrigerate until needed.

Mix soy sauce, cornstarch, salt, and sherry well. Pour over the meat. Mix lightly and let set at room temperature for about ½ hour, or refrigerate for several hours or overnight. Drain well, reserving the marinade.

Spread oil over the bottom of a frying pan. Heat to a frying temperature. Drain the meat well and fry, stirring frequently, until the meat is no longer pink. Add ¼ cup water to the meat along with the reserved marinade. Stir lightly over medium heat.

Add green beans to meat mixture. Cook and stir until beans and meat are both well coated with the sauce. Cover and cook, stirring occasionally, until beans are crisp-tender. Serve about ¾ cup per serving over rice or noodles.

	CAL	CHO (gm)	PRO (gm)	FAT (gm)	NA (mg)
Nutritive values per serving without rice or noodles:	155	10	15	6	927

Food exchanges per serving: 2 vegetables, 2 lean meat
Low-sodium diets: Omit salt and soy sauce.

BEEF MUSHROOM SPAGHETTI SAUCE

Yields 7 cups—14 servings

12 ounces round of beef weighed and ground after fat is removed
1 tablespoon vegetable oil
½ cup finely chopped onions
2 4-ounce cans mushroom stems and pieces
3½ cups (29-ounce can) tomato purée
2 cups tomato juice
2 tablespoons chopped parsley
1 teaspoon salt
½ teaspoon dehydrated garlic
½ teaspoon basil
½ teaspoon leaf oregano
1 teaspoon Italian seasoning

Place beef in a 5- or 6-quart Dutch oven or heavy pot. Cook and stir over moderate heat until it is separated and lightly browned. Place in a strainer and strain off any fat. Set aside to drain. Rinse out the pan with hot water and return it to the heat.

Place oil in Dutch oven. Add onions. Drain mushrooms well. Discard juice and add mushrooms to onions. Cook and stir over moderate heat until onions are soft.

Add remaining ingredients along with meat to onions and mushrooms. Cook over low heat for 30 minutes, stirring frequently. Serve hot over cooked, well-drained spaghetti, ½ cup sauce per serving.

Nutritive values per serving without spaghetti:	CAL	CHO (gm)	PRO (gm)	FAT (gm)	NA (mg)
	74	8	7	3	514

Food exchanges per serving: 1 lean meat, ½ bread
Low-sodium diets: Omit salt. Use low-sodium tomato purée and tomato juice.

STIR-FRY BEEF AND VEGETABLES

Yields 3 cups—3 servings

This stir-fry recipe is an adaptation of a Chinese recipe. Probably no good Chinese cook would recognize it, but we like it and I serve it, or a variation of it, frequently.

8 ounces beef sirloin with fat and gristle removed
¼ cup dry red wine or fat-free beef broth
3 tablespoons soy sauce
1 teaspoon sugar
1½ tablespoons cornstarch
Water
1 tablespoon vegetable oil
2 cups coarsely chopped onions
½ cup thinly sliced celery
½ cup coarsely chopped fresh green peppers
2 tablespoons chopped roasted cashews

Place meat in freezer until it is firm but not frozen. Cut across the grain into bite-size pieces and set aside. Place wine or broth, soy sauce, sugar, and cornstarch in a 2-cup measure. Add enough water to total 1 cup. Stir until smooth and set aside.

Preheat a 10-inch, hard-surface frying pan. (I use a wok frying pan with a T-Fal lining.) Swirl oil around bottom of frying pan, add onions, celery, and green peppers, and cook, stirring frequently, over medium heat until onions are soft but not browned.

Push vegetables to one side of pan, add meat, and cook, stirring the meat frequently, until the meat is rare to well done, as you prefer. Pour wine sauce over meat and vegetables and cook and stir until sauce is clear and thickened. Serve hot over rice or noodles using 1 cup per serving. Garnish each serving with 2 teaspoons of cashews. *Note:* Nutritive information does not include rice or noodles.

Nutritive values per serving:	CAL	CHO (gm)	PRO (gm)	FAT (gm)	NA (mg)
	214	18	15	10	1,079

Food exchanges per serving: 1 bread, 2 lean meat, 1 fat
Low-sodium diets: Use low-sodium soy sauce.

HIGH-FIBER STEW

Yields 6 cups—6 servings

1 pound round of beef or veal weighed after fat and bone are removed
1 tablespoon vegetable oil
3 cups hot fat-free chicken broth
¼ teaspoon thyme
⅛ teaspoon pepper
¼ teaspoon garlic powder
1 teaspoon salt
1 cup carrots cut into 1-inch pieces
4 large stalks celery cut into 1-inch lengths
½ cup coarsely chopped onions
¼ cup chopped fresh green peppers
10-ounce package frozen Brussels sprouts
2 tablespoons cornstarch
¼ cup water

Cut meat into ¾-inch cubes. (This is easier if the meat is slightly frozen.) Place oil on the bottom of a heavy pot. (I use a deep iron frying pan with a glass cover.) Bring to a frying temperature. Add meat and cook, stirring occasionally, until meat is browned and firm.

Add broth and seasonings to meat. Cover and simmer 45 minutes–1 hour or until meat is tender.

Add carrots, celery, onions, and peppers to meat. Cover and simmer 10 minutes. Add Brussels sprouts to stew. Cover and simmer another 12 minutes.

Mix cornstarch and water until smooth. Add to stew and cook and stir until thickened. Continue to simmer for another 2–3 minutes or until starchy taste is gone. Serve hot, 1 cup stew with gravy per serving.

Nutritive values per serving:	CAL	CHO (gm)	PRO (gm)	FAT (gm)	NA (mg)
	177	11	20	6	903

Food exchanges per serving: 2 lean meat, 2 vegetable
Low-sodium diets: Omit salt. Use low-sodium broth.

MARY'S MEATBALLS

Yields 28 meat balls—14 servings

This recipe is based on one from Mary Hinkle here in Wadena. She is my friend Vera Wilson's daughter and a very good cook. I wouldn't dare eat many of her recipes because she makes the very best cookies, cakes, and other desserts and still stays nice and slender—lucky woman!

¼ cup catsup
¼ cup tomato juice
1 tablespoon liquid smoke
½ teaspoon Durkee's barbecue seasoning
1 teaspoon sugar
½ cup oatmeal
¼ cup dry bread crumbs
3 tablespoons grated onions
½ teaspoon salt
¼ teaspoon black pepper
1 cup skim milk
1½ pounds round of beef weighed and ground after fat is removed

Blend first 5 ingredients together well to form a barbecue sauce and set aside at room temperature for later use.

Place oatmeal, crumbs, onions, salt, pepper, and milk in a mixer bowl and mix together at low speed to mix well. Add beef to milk mixture and mix at low speed until blended. Do not overmix. Shape into balls using 2 tablespoons of the mixture for each meatball. Place on a cookie sheet and broil 2–4 minutes. Remove from cookie sheet and place in a casserole, brushing the balls with the barbecue sauce as you put them in the casserole. Pour any remaining sauce over the meatballs, cover, and bake at 325° F. for about 45 minutes or until done. Serve hot, 2 meatballs per serving.

Nutritional values per serving:	CAL	CHO (gm)	PRO (gm)	FAT (gm)	NA (mg)
	98	6	12	3	152

Food exchanges per serving: ½ milk, 1 lean meat
Low-sodium diets: Omit salt. Use low-sodium catsup.

NORWEGIAN MEATBALLS

Yields 18 meatballs—6 servings

This recipe is based on one from Doris Walker of Grinnell, Iowa, who used to live in Wadena when we first moved here.

2 tablespoons cornstarch
¾ teaspoon salt
½ teaspoon nutmeg
2 large egg whites
¾ cup skim milk
1 pound ground round of beef weighed and ground after fat is removed
⅔ cup Campbell's Cream of Mushroom soup

Place first 4 ingredients and ¼ cup of the milk in mixer bowl and mix at low speed to blend well. Add beef to mixer bowl and mix at low speed to blend well. Shape 18 meatballs using about 1½ tablespoons mix per meatball. (The mixture will be soft.) Place in a 9" × 13" cake pan that has been lined with aluminum foil or sprayed with pan spray. Bake 30 minutes at 375° F. Remove from pan while still hot and place in a 1½-quart casserole.

Mix soup and remaining ½ cup milk well and pour over meatballs. Cover and bake at 350° F. for 30 minutes. Serve 3 meatballs per serving with a little of the sauce.

Nutritive values per serving:	CAL	CHO (gm)	PRO (gm)	FAT (gm)	NA (mg)
	148	6	19	5	464

Food exchanges per serving: 1 vegetable, 2 lean meat
Low-sodium diets: Omit salt. Use low-sodium soup.

CHICAGO CHILI

Yields 6 cups—6 servings

This is the recipe Chuck developed when he owned a restaurant in Chicago. He always served it in a bowl with the beans on the side. If you add canned beans to your chili, add 1 bread exchange for each ½ cup hot, cooked, drained kidney or pinto beans that you stir into a bowl of chili.

1 tablespoon vegetable oil
1 cup chopped onions
1 pound ground round of beef weighed and ground after bone and fat
   are removed
2 cups chopped solid-pack canned tomatoes with juice
1 cup tomato purée
1 cup tomato juice
3 cups fat-free chicken broth
1 teaspoon sugar
1½ teaspoons salt
¼ teaspoon pepper
½ teaspoon garlic powder
¼ teaspoon ground cumin
½ teaspoon ground oregano
1 teaspoon chili powder

Pour the oil into a heavy pot. Bring to frying temperature over moderate heat. Add the onions and cook and stir over moderate heat until onions are soft but not golden.

Add beef to onions. Cook and stir over moderate heat until meat is well browned and broken into small pieces. Pour meat and onions into a colander and drain off any fat and liquid. Discard fat and liquid, rinse the pot out with hot water, and then return the meat and onions to the pot.

Add remaining ingredients to meat mixture. Bring to a boil, reduce heat, and simmer, uncovered, for 1¼ hours, stirring occasionally. Serve hot using 1 cup chili per serving.

Nutritive values per serving:

	CAL	CHO (gm)	PRO (gm)	FAT (gm)	NA (mg)
	178	12	19	6	1,356

Food exchanges per serving: 2 vegetable, 2 lean meat
Low-sodium diets: Omit salt. Use low-sodium tomatoes, tomato purée, tomato juice, and chicken broth.

BARBECUE MEAT LOAF

Yields 1 loaf—6 servings

¼ **cup finely chopped onions**
¼ **cup finely chopped celery**
¼ **cup catsup**
2 large egg whites
¼ **cup dry bread crumbs**
1 teaspoon liquid smoke
1 teaspoon salt
¹⁄₁₆ **teaspoon black pepper**
1 pound round of beef weighed and ground after fat is removed

Place all ingredients except beef in mixer bowl and mix at low speed to blend well.

Add beef to catsup mixture and mix at low speed until blended. Do not overmix. Shape into a loaf about 3½″ × 7″. Place in a pan that has been sprayed with pan spray or lined with aluminum foil. Bake at 325° F. about 1 hour or until browned and firm. Pour off any fat and drippings and let set for 10 minutes before cutting into 6 equal slices. Serve 1 slice per serving.

Nutritional values per serving:	CAL	CHO (gm)	PRO (gm)	FAT (gm)	NA (mg)
	138	6	17	4	513

Food exchanges per serving: 2 lean meat, 1 vegetable
Low-sodium diets: Omit salt. Use low-sodium catsup.

MEAT LOAF WITH FIBER

Yields 1 loaf—8 servings

1 cup All-Bran, Bran Buds, or 100% Bran
¼ cup finely chopped onions
3 large egg whites
1 cup tomato sauce
1 teaspoon Worcestershire sauce
1 teaspoon dry mustard
½ teaspoon salt
¹⁄₁₆ teaspoon pepper
1 pound 4 ounces round of beef weighed and ground after fat is
removed

Place all ingredients except beef in mixer bowl and mix at low speed to blend.

Add beef to bran mixture and blend at low speed. Do not overmix. Shape into a loaf and place in a pan that has been sprayed with pan spray or lined with aluminum foil. Bake at 325° F. about 1¼ hours or until browned and firm. Pour off any fat and drippings and let set for 10 minutes. Cut into 8 equal slices. Serve 1 slice per serving.

Nutritive values per serving:	CAL	CHO (gm)	PRO (gm)	FAT (gm)	NA (mg)
	163	9	17	6	213

Food exchanges per serving: ½ bread, 2 lean meat
Low-sodium diets: Omit salt and Worcestershire sauce. Add ½ teaspoon basil along with pepper.

BAKED PORK AND RICE

Yields about 3 cups—4 servings

12-ounces pork tenderloin weighed after visible fat is removed
1 cup thinly sliced celery
½ cup chopped onions
1½ cups fat-free chicken broth
½ cup long-grain rice
2 tablespoons soy sauce
Whisper of black pepper
3 tablespoons chopped pimientos

Cut pork into ½-inch cubes. Place in a shallow pan and bake at 350° F. about 30 minutes or until browned. Remove from pan with a slotted spoon and place in a 1½-quart casserole. .

Place celery, onions, and broth in a small saucepan. Bring to a boil, reduce heat, cover, and simmer for 10 minutes. Add rice, soy sauce, and pepper to hot broth. Mix lightly and add to meat in casserole. Mix lightly. Cover tightly and bake at 350° F. about 40 minutes or until rice is tender. Remove from oven.

Stir pimientos into hot pork and rice. Serve hot, using ¼ of the total (about ¾ cup) per serving.

Nutritive values per serving:	CAL	CHO (gm)	PRO (gm)	FAT (gm)	NA (mg)
	212	23	20	7	1,213

Food exchanges per serving: 1½ bread, 2 lean meat
Low-sodium diets: Omit soy sauce. Use low-sodium chicken broth.

SWEET SOUR PORK

Yields 5 cups—5 servings

**1 pound lean pork from fresh ham or tenderloin weighed after bone and
  fat are removed**
1 tablespoon vegetable oil
2 cups fat-free chicken broth
1½ cups thinly sliced celery
½ cup coarsely chopped onions
¼ cup soy sauce
2 tablespoons cornstarch
⅓ cup vinegar
¼-⅓ cup Brown Sugar Twin granulated sugar substitute
1 large tomato cut into wedges
1 cup drained, canned unsweetened pineapple tidbits

Cut pork into small pieces about 1" × ¼". (It is easier to cut the pork this
thin if it is slightly frozen.) Place oil in the bottom of a heavy frying pan or
saucepan. Bring to frying temperature. Add pork and cook and stir over
moderate heat until pork is browned and cooked. Remove pork with slotted
spoon and set aside for later use. Pour off as much of the fat as possible
from the pan and then blot up any remaining fat with a paper towel.

Add broth to frying pan. Cook and stir over low heat to get up the
browned bits in the bottom of the pan. Add celery and onions to hot
chicken broth. Cover and simmer 10 minutes.

Mix soy sauce, cornstarch, and vinegar until smooth. Add to vegetables
and cook and stir over moderate heat until thickened. Add sweetener to
vegetables to taste and mix lightly.

Add tomatoes and pineapple to vegetables along with the pork. Cook
over low heat until serving temperature, stirring occasionally. Do not allow
to boil. The tomato wedges should be hot but not cooked. Serve hot over
cooked rice using 1 cup per serving.

Nutritive values per serving without rice:	CAL	CHO (gm)	PRO (gm)	FAT (gm)	NA (mg)
	188	15	16	8	1,521

Food exchanges per serving: 1 bread, 2 lean meat
Low-sodium diets: This recipe is not suitable.

PAN GRAVY

Yields 2 cups—8 servings

This gravy is a great favorite in the Midwest. It is served often and in large quantities. I have never lived down the time we were visiting my cousin Virginia Ballantine in Clarion, Iowa, when we were still living in Chicago. She was busy getting dinner and asked me to make the gravy. I made about this much, which is what I make at home. When her husband and two grown sons looked at that tiny bowl of gravy—well, you wouldn't believe how they teased me about starving them, and city cooks, and above all dietitians! I'm still hearing about it years later, even though I have made it in larger quantities for them many times since then.

1 tablespoon vegetable oil
¼ cup all-purpose flour
2½ cups cold water
½ teaspoon salt
Whisper of pepper

Pour all of the fat out of a pan in which you have pan-fried steak, chicken, pork chops, or other meats. Blot out remaining fat with a paper towel. Add the oil to the pan and bring the pan to a frying temperature. Add flour to oil and cook and stir until browned and smooth.

Add the water to the flour mixture; cook and stir over moderate heat until thickened and you have scraped all of the brown bits from the pan. Add salt and pepper to the gravy. Mix lightly and serve hot, using ¼ cup gravy per serving.

Nutritive values per serving:	CAL	CHO (gm)	PRO (gm)	FAT (gm)	NA (mg)
	29	3	negl.	2	133

Food exchanges per serving: ½ vegetable
Low-sodium diets: Omit salt.

BROWN GRAVY

Yields 2 cups—8 servings

The flavor of this gravy depends upon the flavor of the drippings or broth that you use as a base. It can be luscious or it can be blah. I prefer to use drippings from roasts. I chill them and remove the fat and the murky stuff at the bottom and then save them for gravy.

2¼ cups cold fat-free drippings or broth
2 tablespoons cornstarch
Whisper of pepper
½ teaspoon Kitchen Bouquet
Salt to taste

Place drippings, cornstarch, and pepper in a small saucepan and mix together until smooth. Place over moderate heat and cook and stir until smooth and thickened, using a wire whisk. Taste for flavoring and add salt and Kitchen Bouquet if necessary. Serve hot, using ¼ cup per serving.

Nutritive values per serving:	CAL	CHO (gm)	PRO (gm)	FAT (gm)	NA (mg)
	9	2	negl.	negl.	*

Food exchanges per serving: ¼ cup may be considered free
Low-sodium diets: Omit salt. Use salt-free broth or drippings.

*varies with amount used

BROWN RICE DRESSING

Yields 6 cups—12 servings

1 cup raw brown rice
2½ cups fat-free chicken broth
1 tablespoon vegetable oil
2 cups thinly sliced celery
1 cup chopped onions
1 4-ounce can drained mushroom stems and pieces
1 8-ounce can water chestnuts
½ teaspoon leaf thyme
½ teaspoon rosemary
¹⁄₁₆ teaspoon black pepper
¼ teaspoon salt
½ teaspoon sage

Combine rice and broth in a saucepan. Heat to boiling. Stir, cover, and reduce heat. Simmer 45–50 minutes or until tender.

Place oil in saucepan. Bring to frying temperature. Add celery, onions, and mushrooms to hot oil. Cook, stirring frequently, over moderate heat, until onions are just tender. Drain chestnuts well. Slice into thin slices and add to hot vegetables.

Add remaining seasonings to vegetables and cook over low heat for 4 minutes, stirring frequently. Add rice and toss lightly. Reheat, if necessary, stirring gently over low heat. Serve hot using ½ cup per serving.

Nutritive values per serving:	CAL	CHO (gm)	PRO (gm)	FAT (gm)	NA (mg)
	88	17	2	2	353

Food exchanges per serving: 1 bread
Low-sodium diets: Omit salt. Use low-sodium broth.

11
VEGETABLES, ETC.

There is such an abundance of interesting fresh, frozen, dried, and canned vegetables available these days that we shouldn't ever complain that we don't know what vegetable to have for dinner that day. They can be prepared very simply or they can be the star of the menu—and you can eat your fill of vegetables without adding all that much carbohydrate to the meal. Vegetables don't contain any cholesterol so we should really appreciate them from both the low-cholesterol and the low-calorie viewpoints.

Vegetables contain a great deal of fiber, vitamins, and minerals; they even have a little protein, although only a trace of fat. They also taste delicious, which is a definite plus.

Vegetables fresh from the garden are wonderful in the summer. I always enjoy seeing how much Frances Nielsen and Chuck relish fresh vegetables. Both of them are so pleased with the first ripe tomato, the first fresh green beans, those little potatoes fresh from the garden and the green onions. Chuck grows more onions than anyone else because both Frances and I dote on those little green onions.

If you can't get vegetables fresh from the garden, frozen ones are next best. Sometimes frozen vegetables can be even better than fresh because they are picked and frozen at the peak of their perfection (and haven't stayed in the refrigerator until you get around to using them as they do in my house sometimes).

It is best to use fresh or frozen vegetables on a low-sodium diet because most canned vegetables have salt added to them when they are processed. If you can't get either fresh or frozen vegetables for your low-sodium diet, drain the liquid off the vegetables (except for tomatoes or some other vegetable where the liquid is important) and replace it with water. This will lower the sodium content somewhat. There are also vegetables available now that are canned without added salt, and they are a good buy on a low-sodium diet—or you can can your own vegetables (see Chapter 18) without adding any salt when you process them.

If you aren't on a low-sodium diet, canned vegetables are an excellent source of fiber, vitamins, and minerals. There is such a variety of them and they are always available. We like to keep a good supply of them on hand in our fruit room so we have them when we want them. If you do keep some canned vegetables on hand, they should be kept in a cool place (around 70° F. or lower), out of direct light, and should be rotated. Use the oldest cans first. In fact, Chuck dates the cans of vegetables as we buy them so we will know which should be used first. It is disconcerting to discover some canned vegetables a couple of years old that got shoved to the back of the shelf and not used when they were fresh.

If the cans show any signs of spoilage they should be discarded. If they are bulging or leaking or have a bad smell when you open them, discard them immediately. Don't ever taste them to see if they are good. Just tasting them, if there is botulism in the cans, can cause death. Very few cases of botulism have been reported in this country in this century, but it still pays to be cautious.

Although many vegetables are very low in carbohydrate, some vegetables are higher in carbohydrate and need to be included under the bread exchanges on a diabetic diet. I would have liked to have included more beans, brown rice, peas, and other starchy vegetables in this chapter because of their good fiber content; however, we will get sufficient fiber in our diet if we eat a good supply of the other vegetables. Most dietitians will tell you that if you eat whole wheat bread, an occasional special bran bread or muffin, and four or more servings of fruits and vegetables daily, you will get enough fiber.

I do enjoy beans in any form. I usually consider them a special treat that I can have when the carbohydrate content of my meal is very low—or I use a couple of tablespoons of them in a lettuce salad to add interest to the salad (2 tablespoons of baked beans is 1 vegetable exchange). If you have a liberal diabetic diet and can afford it, I highly recommend that you use a good quantity of beans and other starchy vegetables because of their taste and good fiber content.

All of our diabetic lists include the values for vegetables, so I haven't included many plain vegetables in this chapter. I have tried to show you how to add a little zing to a few of them. I hope you'll try them, and perhaps adapt some of your own vegetable recipes using the information in Chapter 2, "Calculating Food Exchanges," and also develop some of your own special recipes.

GREEN BEAN AND MUSHROOM CASSEROLE

Yields 4 cups—4 servings

This recipe was given to me by M. J. Smith, a registered dietitian from Guttenberg, Iowa. She is an innovative dietitian who sends subscribers a monthly menu plan complete with menus, recipes, a shopping list, and current information on nutrition and new foods available in the marketplace. She calls her service Menu Management, Inc., and it is a great help for those who want interesting, low-calorie menus and recipes without having to do all of the research involved.

1 10-ounce package frozen French-cut green beans
1 teaspoon liquid margarine
8 ounces fresh mushrooms, sliced
½ cup plain low-fat yogurt
1 tablespoon all-purpose flour
1 tablespoon dry sherry
2 teaspoons Worcestershire sauce

Thaw green beans. Preheat a small, hard-surface, nonstick frying pan over medium heat for 1 minute. Swirl margarine in it, add mushrooms, and cook and stir over medium heat until mushrooms are tender.

Combine yogurt, flour, sherry, and Worcestershire sauce in a 1½-quart casserole and stir until smooth. Fold mushrooms and beans into sauce and bake at 350° F. for 35–40 minutes. Serve hot, using 1 cup per serving.

Nutritive values per serving:	CAL	CHO (gm)	PRO (gm)	FAT (gm)	NA (mg)
	103	7	4	3	95

Food exchanges per serving: ½ bread, ½ fat
Low-sodium diets: May be used as written.

CREOLE GREEN BEANS

Yields 4 cups—8 servings

1 tablespoon vegetable oil
¼ cup chopped onions
¼ cup thinly sliced celery
1 tablespoon flour
1 cup tomato juice
¼ teaspoon salt
Whisper of pepper
2 16-ounce cans green string beans

Place oil in a saucepan and heat to frying temperature over moderate heat. Add onions and celery to oil and cook and stir over moderate heat until the onions are soft but not browned. Add flour to vegetables and cook and stir until the flour is absorbed by the vegetables. Add tomato juice, salt, and pepper to the vegetables and cook and stir over moderate heat until slightly thickened and smooth.

Drain beans well. Add to hot sauce and simmer 2 minutes over moderate heat. Serve hot, using ½ cup per serving.

Nutritive values per serving:	CAL	CHO (gm)	PRO (gm)	FAT (gm)	NA (mg)
	48	8	2	2	415

Food exchanges per serving: ½ bread
Low-sodium diets: Omit salt. Wash green beans well with cold water after they are drained. Drain well again and add to sauce.

BROCCOLI RICE CASSEROLE

Yields 5 cups—10 servings

1 tablespoon vegetable oil
1 cup chopped onions
1 pound fresh or frozen broccoli pieces
1 can cream of mushroom soup
¼ cup milk
1 cup cooked rice
2 tablespoons grated Parmesan cheese

Place oil in a saucepan and bring to a frying temperature. Add onions to oil and cook and stir over moderate heat until soft but not browned. Add broccoli to onions and cook and stir over moderate heat until hot but not cooked. Mix soup and milk together to blend and add to broccoli mixture.

Add rice to vegetables. Cook and stir over low heat until hot and mixed. Place in a 1½- or 2-quart casserole that has been greased with margarine.

Sprinkle Parmesan evenly over the top of the broccoli mixture. Bake, uncovered, at 350° F. for 35–40 minutes or until the casserole is bubbly and the broccoli is cooked. Serve hot using ½ cup per serving.

Nutritive values per serving:	CAL	CHO (gm)	PRO (gm)	FAT (gm)	NA (mg)
	67	9	3	3	246

Food exchanges per serving: 2 vegetables, 1 fat
Low-sodium diets: Cook rice without salt and use low-sodium soup.

CHINESE VEGETABLES

Yields 3 cups—6 servings

We like this served as a vegetable with plain roast pork or baked chicken. My sister says it tastes like chop suey and I guess she is right—but I like chop suey very much so that doesn't bother me.

1 tablespoon vegetable oil
½ cup coarsely chopped onions
1 cup thinly sliced celery
1 4-ounce can of well-drained mushrooms
1 cup water
1½ tablespoons cornstarch
¼ cup soy sauce
1 14-ounce can of well-drained bean sprouts
2 tablespoons chopped cashew nuts roasted in oil

Place oil in a saucepan and bring to a frying temperature. Add onions, celery, and mushrooms to hot oil. Cook and stir over moderate heat for 2–3 minutes or until onions are softened. Add ¼ cup water to vegetables. Cover and cook over low heat about 8 minutes or until vegetables are tender.

Mix together ¾ cup water, cornstarch, and soy sauce until smooth. Add to vegetables and cook and stir over moderate heat until thickened and clear. Add sprouts and nuts to vegetables and heat to serving temperature. Serve hot using ½ cup per serving.

Nutritive values per serving:

	CAL	CHO (gm)	PRO (gm)	FAT (gm)	NA (mg)
	68	7	3	4	975

Food exchanges per serving: 1 vegetable, 1 fat
Low-sodium diets: This recipe is not suitable.

SHREDDED CABBAGE

Yields 2 cups—4 servings

1 pound white cabbage
¼ cup water
½ teaspoon salt
1 tablespoon margarine
Dash of pepper

Trim and wash cabbage. Shred coarsely or cut into slices about ⅛ inch wide. Place water and salt in a saucepan and bring to a boil. Add cabbage. Mix lightly and cover tightly. Simmer over low heat for 12 minutes, stirring once during the cooking period. Drain well. Add margarine and pepper to cabbage. Toss lightly and serve hot, using ½ cup cabbage per serving.

Nutritive values per serving:	CAL	CHO (gm)	PRO (gm)	FAT (gm)	NA (mg)
	53	6	2	3	324

Food exchanges per serving: 1 vegetable, ½ fat
Low-sodium diets: Omit salt.

CAULIFLOWER PARMESAN

Yields about 2 cups—4 servings

Chuck's cousin Dave Cavaiani's wife Etta cooked this for us when we visited them in Iron Mountain and we really liked it. The cheese adds to the flavor of the cauliflower in a most attractive way.

1 pound frozen cauliflower
2 cups boiling water
1 teaspoon salt
1 tablespoon margarine
2 tablespoons grated Parmesan cheese

Place cauliflower, water, and salt in a saucepan, cover, and simmer about 8 minutes or until the cauliflower is tender; or cook in the microwave oven according to directions on the package. Drain well.

Sprinkle margarine and cheese over the cauliflower. Toss lightly to coat the cauliflower and serve hot, using ¼ of the cauliflower (about ½ cup) per serving.

Nutritive values per serving:	CAL	CHO (gm)	PRO (gm)	FAT (gm)	NA (mg)
	68	6	4	4	605

Food exchanges per serving: 1 vegetable, 1 fat
Low-sodium diets: Omit salt.

EGGPLANT AND TOMATOES

Yields 6 cups—12 servings

1 1-pound eggplant
¼ cup vegetable oil
½ cup coarsely chopped onions
½ cup coarsely chopped fresh green peppers
1 finely minced garlic clove
2 cups (1-pound can) Italian plum tomatoes
¼ cup chopped fresh parsley
⅛ teaspoon pepper
1 teaspoon salt
1 teaspoon sugar

Wash eggplant and remove ends. Cut into ½-inch cubes without removing the skin. Place oil in the bottom of a heavy pot or frying pan. Add eggplant along with onions, peppers, and garlic and fry over moderate heat, stirring occasionally, until eggplant is transparent and tender.

Add remaining ingredients to eggplant mixture and cook, stirring frequently, over moderate heat for about 5 minutes. Serve hot or at room temperature, using ½ cup per serving.

Nutritive values per serving:	CAL	CHO (gm)	PRO (gm)	FAT (gm)	NA (mg)
	63	5	1	5	231

Food exchanges per serving: 1 vegetable, 1 fat
Low-sodium diets: Omit salt. Use low-sodium canned tomatoes or fresh tomatoes.

SAUERKRAUT WITH TOMATOES

Yields 1 quart—8 servings

I wish you could meet Dave Christen, who gave me this recipe. To me, he represents all the best in small-town residents. He truly cares about the town and his neighbors. He is a quiet family man who enjoys cooking occasionally. He and his wife, Dorothy, are active in their church and in the First Responders, who quickly arrive in an emergency in a small town. He is commander of his American Legion Post, is active in the fire department, and last year was president of his state professional organization, the Iowa Blacksmith and Welder's Association.

1 29-ounce can sauerkraut
1 16-ounce can whole tomatoes with juice
½ cup cooked, diced, very lean ham with all visible fat removed
½ cup chopped onions
2 tablespoons packed brown sugar
½ teaspoon brown Sweet'n Low sugar substitute

Place sauerkraut in a colander, rinse with 2 quarts cold water, and drain well. Place sauerkraut in a large bowl, add tomatoes and juice, ham, onions, and brown sugar, and mix well. Place in a 2-quart casserole. Cover and bake at 325° F. for 1 hour.

Remove cover, stir lightly, and bake 1 more hour. (Dave says he sometimes does this in a Crockpot for picnics.) Stir sugar substitute into sauerkraut mixture and serve hot, using ½ cup per serving.

Nutritive values per serving:	CAL	CHO (gm)	PRO (gm)	FAT (gm)	NA (mg)
	63	10	4	2	313

Food exchanges per serving: 2 vegetable
Low-sodium diets: Use low-sodium tomatoes and rinse and drain sauerkraut well.

PICKLED VEGETABLES

Yields about 1 gallon—32 servings

These vegetables can be canned but I never bother to do so. I prepare them one recipe at a time and keep them in the refrigerator where they keep well for several weeks.

3 cups vinegar
3 cups water
3 tablespoons pickling spices
1 pound fresh carrots
1 10-ounce package frozen Brussels sprouts
2 cups celery cut into thin slices
2 cups (1-pound can) drained canned green beans
2 cups (1-pound can) drained canned yellow wax beans
2 cups julienne-cut fresh green peppers
2 cups coarsely chopped onions
Sugar substitute equal to 2 cups sugar

Combine vinegar, water, and pickling spices in a saucepan. Bring to a boil and simmer, covered, for 3 minutes. Remove from heat, cover, and let stand at room temperature for about a week or until the vinegar mixture tastes spicy according to your taste. Discard spices.

Clean carrots and cut into julienne pieces. Combine carrots, Brussels sprouts, and celery. Cover with boiling water and cook 3 minutes. Remove from heat; drain. Cover with cold water and drain again. Place in a large kettle with the vinegar mixture. Drain beans well and add to carrot and vinegar mixture.

Add peppers and onions to vegetables. Bring to a boil but remove immediately from heat. The vegetables should not be allowed to boil. Add sweetener to vegetable mixture. Mix lightly. Cover and allow to come to room temperature. Refrigerate at least 3 days before serving (½ cup per serving) as a salad or vegetable.

Nutritive values per serving:	CAL	CHO (gm)	PRO (gm)	FAT (gm)	NA (mg)
	26	6	1	negl.	90
Food exchanges per serving:	1 vegetable (up to 3 tablespoons may be considered free)				
Low-sodium diets:	Omit canned beans. Use 2 pounds frozen green or wax beans that have been cooked without salt.				

SOUTHERN-STYLE GREENS

Yields about 2 cups—4 servings

1 pound frozen mustard or turnip greens
4 ounces chopped center-cut ham with fat, bone, and skin removed
¹/₁₆ teaspoon black pepper
1½ cups boiling water

Greens should be almost completely thawed before cooking. Place greens in a saucepan. Add ham, pepper, and water to greens. Bring to a boil, reduce heat, and simmer uncovered for 30 minutes or until tender, adding more hot water if necessary. Cut through the greens several times with a sharp knife. Serve hot with some of the juice using ½ cup greens per serving.

Nutritive values per serving:

	CAL	CHO (gm)	PRO (gm)	FAT (gm)	NA (mg)
	99	4	7	7	258

Food exchanges per serving: 1 vegetable, 1 lean meat, 1 fat
Low-sodium diets: May be used as written.

SPINACH FRITATTA

Yields 1 fritatta—1 serving

I'm very fond of fritattas and make them frequently. I use a variety of vegetables, and sometimes I use ¼ cup cooked rice instead of bread.

2½ ounces frozen chopped spinach
¼ cup finely chopped onions
1 tablespoon imitation bacon bits
⅛ teaspoon salt
Sprinkle of pepper
Whites from 2 large or 3 medium eggs
½ slice whole wheat bread cut into cubes
½ teaspoon margarine

Cut a 10-ounce package of frozen chopped spinach into quarters. Defrost one quarter and return the rest to the freezer. Press any liquid out of spinach. Put spinach into a small bowl with onions, bacon bits, salt, pepper, and egg whites. Mix well with a fork. Add bread cubes and mix lightly, until they are covered with egg mixture but not soaked.

Preheat an 8-inch hard-surface, nonstick frying pan over medium heat for 1 minute. Swirl margarine around bottom of pan. Add spinach mixture and fry over medium heat until bottom is lightly browned. Turn fritatta over and cook until firm and bottom is lightly browned. Serve hot, using 1 fritatta per serving. *Note:* If you want to make several fritattas, it is best to make them individually.

Nutritive values per serving:	CAL	CHO (gm)	PRO (gm)	FAT (gm)	NA (mg)
	126	14	12	3	571

Food exchanges per serving: 1 bread, 1 lean meat
Low-sodium diets: Omit salt.

SUMMER SQUASH WITH GINGER

Yields 3 cups—6 servings

I've never cared much for summer squash but when Chef Dave Hutchins served this to us at a luncheon, I knew I had finally found a recipe for summer squash I could enjoy. He is a very interesting person with an excellent professional background. His extensive knowledge about food and its preparation is reflected in the wonderful and varied food he serves in his restaurant. Chuck and I love to talk to him and his wife Alice when we go there for dinner.

1 tablespoon vegetable oil
3 cups ¼-inch slices of summer squash (about 6 small zucchini)
1½ teaspoons finely chopped fresh ginger
4 crushed garlic cloves
1 cup peeled, seeded, and chopped fresh tomatoes
1 teaspoon grated Parmesan cheese
½ teaspoon salt
Sprinkle of pepper

Preheat a 12-inch hard-surface, nonstick frying pan. Swirl oil around pan, add squash, ginger, and garlic, and cook, stirring frequently, until squash is soft but not transparent. Add tomato to the sauce and continue to cook over medium heat, stirring frequently, until squash is transparent. Stir in Parmesan, salt, and pepper. Serve hot, using ½ cup per serving.

Nutritive values per serving:	CAL	CHO (gm)	PRO (gm)	FAT (gm)	NA (mg)
	50	5	2	3	189

Food exchanges per serving: 1 vegetable, 1 fat
Low-sodium diets: Omit salt.

MONK'S RICE

Yields 5 cups—10 servings

Margaret "Monk" Sellers prepared this rice when we both visited her sister and brother-in-law, Frances and Bud Gunsallus, in Miami. Monk said that she likes this version because the rice and vegetables aren't soupy or gummy as they are when you cook them all in the same pot. She prepared a big roaster full of it for the family party that night and we ate every bite of it.

½ **cup long-grain rice**
1 **cup chicken broth**
1 **tablespoon vegetable oil**
2 **cups broccoli ends and pieces**
1 **cup coarsely chopped onions**
1 **cup coarsely grated carrots**
½ **cup chopped fresh green peppers**
½ **cup thinly sliced celery**
1 **4-ounce can well-drained mushroom stems and pieces**
¼ **teaspoon salt**

Combine rice and broth and bring to a boil. Pour in a small casserole, cover tightly, and bake at 350° F. for 30 minutes. Remove cover and set aside for later use.

Spread oil in a heavy 9- or 10-inch frying pan. Bring to a cooking temperature over moderate heat.

Add vegetables and salt to hot oil in frying pan. Cook, stirring frequently, over moderate heat 10–15 minutes or until vegetables are crisp-tender (or soft if you prefer them that way). Add rice and mix lightly. Serve ½ cup per serving.

Nutritive values per serving:	CAL	CHO (gm)	PRO (gm)	FAT (gm)	NA (mg)
	70	12	2	2	209

Food exchanges per serving: 1 vegetable, ½ bread
Low-sodium diets: Omit salt. Use low-sodium chicken broth.

SAUTÉED VEGETABLES

Yields 3 cups—6 servings

2 teaspoons vegetable oil
2 cups coarsely shredded cabbage
1 cup coarsely shredded carrots
1½ cups thinly sliced celery
¼ cup chopped fresh green peppers
½ cup coarsely chopped onions
½ teaspoon salt
¼ cup water
Soy sauce as desired

Place oil in the bottom of a heavy saucepan and heat to frying temperature. Add vegetables and salt to oil. Cook over moderate heat for 5 minutes, stirring frequently.

Add ¼ cup water to vegetables, cover, and cook over low heat for 5–7 minutes or until vegetables have reached the desired tenderness. Serve vegetables hot, using ½ cup per serving, with soy sauce to be added as desired.

Nutritive values per serving without soy sauce:	CAL	CHO (gm)	PRO (gm)	FAT (gm)	NA (mg)
	35	5	1	2	384

Food exchanges per serving: 1 vegetable
Low-sodium diets: Omit salt. Do not use soy sauce.

BAKED TOMATO HALVES

Yields 8 halves—4 servings

Frances Nielsen taught me to make these when she lived here in Wadena. The tomatoes are best right out of the garden. They should be fully ripe but still firm. The seasoning can be varied using basil, oregano, or any other favorite seasoning instead of the garlic.

4 fresh, ripe, medium-size tomatoes
2 tablespoons melted margarine
1 teaspoon garlic salt
1/16 teaspoon pepper
4 teaspoons grated Parmesan cheese
2 teaspoons dried parsley flakes

Wash tomatoes and remove the stems. Cut the tomatoes in half crosswise and place the halves on a rimmed cookie sheet that has been greased with margarine or sprayed with pan spray. Brush the tomato halves with margarine using a pastry brush.

Sprinkle the garlic salt and pepper on the tops of the tomato halves and then sprinkle the halves with the Parmesan cheese and parsley flakes, using ½ teaspoon of cheese for each tomato half. Bake at 350° F. for 35–45 minutes or until tender and lightly browned. Serve hot using 2 halves per serving.

Nutritive values per serving:	CAL	CHO (gm)	PRO (gm)	FAT (gm)	NA (mg)
	87	6	2	6	489

Food exchanges per serving: 1 vegetable, 1 fat
Low-sodium diets: Omit salt.

STIR-FRY TOMATOES

Yields about 6 cups—8 servings

1 tablespoon vegetable oil
1 cup thinly sliced celery
1 cup julienne-cut fresh green peppers
1 6- to 8-inch zucchini cut into ¼-inch slices
4 medium-size tomatoes at room temperature
1 cup fat-free chicken broth
1 tablespoon cornstarch
¼ teaspoon salt
½ teaspoon ground ginger
1¹/₁₆ teaspoons pepper

Place oil in heavy saucepan or deep, heavy frying pan and bring to frying temperature. Add celery, peppers, and zucchini to frying pan. Cook and stir over moderate heat about 5 minutes, or until crisp-tender. Wash tomatoes and remove stems. Cut into wedges and add to vegetable mixture. Cook and stir until tomatoes are hot.

Stir together broth, cornstarch, and seasonings until smooth. Add to vegetables and cook and stir about 2 minutes or until thickened. Serve hot using about ¾ cup per serving.

Nutritive values per serving:

CAL	CHO (gm)	PRO (gm)	FAT (gm)	NA (mg)
42	6	1	2	210

Food exchanges per serving: 1 vegetable
Low-sodium diets: Omit salt. Use low-sodium broth.

ZUCCHINI SCRAMBLE

Yields about 4 cups—8 servings

My sister-in-law, Josephine Severino of Chicago, says this is one of her favorite summer vegetable combinations.

1 tablespoon vegetable oil
1 6- to 8-inch zucchini cut into ¼-inch slices
1 cup fresh green peppers cut into thin julienne strips
½ cup diced fresh potatoes
½ cup coarsely chopped onions
1 large fresh tomato cut into wedges
¼ teaspoon garlic powder
½ teaspoon salt
1 bay leaf

Place oil in a heavy saucepan or deep, heavy frying pan and bring to frying temperature.

Add vegetables and seasonings to hot oil. Cook and stir over moderate heat for about 3 minutes. Reduce heat to low, cover, and cook, stirring occasionally, about 20 minutes or until vegetables are tender. Remove bay leaf and serve hot, using about ½ cup per portion.

Nutritive values per serving:	CAL	CHO (gm)	PRO (gm)	FAT (gm)	NA (mg)
	39	5	1	2	137

Food exchanges per serving: 1 vegetable
Low-sodium diets: Omit salt.

VEGETABLE PURÉES

This is a method, not a recipe, but I urge you to try it. The vegetable purées are very flavorful and attractive—a whole new taste sensation. Since they are more concentrated than the regular vegetables, ⅓ of a cup of puréed vegetable is equal to ½ cup of the same vegetable—but it is worth it. I add margarine and other seasonings after the vegetables are puréed, except for the salt that I add when cooking the vegetable. If you add 1 tablespoon of margarine per cup of cooked puréed vegetables, you will have 1 vegetable exchange and 1 fat exchange per ⅓ cup of puréed vegetable.

Start with good fresh vegetables. Wash them, and peel them if necessary. Cook them until tender but not mushy. I prefer to cook vegetables in the microwave, but you can also cook them in water if you prefer. If you have cooked them in water, drain them well and shake the pan over low heat for a few seconds to get rid of as much moisture as possible. If you have cooked them in the microwave, drain them well and cover them with a clean napkin or dishtowel for a few minutes to absorb as much of the steam as possible.

Vegetables can be sieved or put into the food processor. I prefer the food processor because it is much simpler. I don't recommend the blender because you have to add a little water and the results aren't firm enough. Remove any seeds or skin you don't want to be in the purée before you put the food in the food processor because it will process everything together.

The vegetable purée will probably be cold after it is finished. I add seasonings then along with the margarine. The purée can be reheated by placing it in the microwave, or it can be stirred over low heat in a saucepan until it is at serving temperature. If I'm having guests, I like to put it in a casserole and put it in the oven to be lightly browned before it is served. You can also freeze the purées in ⅓ cup portions to add interest to some other meals in the future. If you do this, it is better not to add the margarine until you are ready to defrost and reheat the vegetables.

Potatoes should not be prepared in the food processor because the action of the food processor will make the potatoes gummy. However, winter squash and carrots both react well in the food processor. I also like to combine vegetables, puréeing them separately or together, such as adding onions to winter squash or broccoli, or a little green pepper to carrots. One of my favorites is to add some dill seed to puréed winter squash. There are so many good combinations to explore that your vegetable exchanges should never be dull.

BAKED BEANS

Yields 6 cups—18 servings

These are my sister Shirley's favorite. I wish I could use more of them in my diet because I also like them and they are a good source of fiber, but they are so high in carbohydrate that I don't use them too often. Some-times I add a couple of tablespoons of them to a big lettuce salad—which is very good and only costs me a vegetable exchange.

1 pound dry great northern beans
Cold water as necessary
4 ounces chopped center-cut ham with fat, bone, and skin removed
1 cup chopped onions
6 ounces tomato paste
1½ teaspoons salt
2 tablespoons salad mustard
¾ cup Brown Sugar Twin granulated sugar substitute

Wash beans and discard any imperfect ones. Add cold water, cover, and bring to a boil. Simmer for 5 minutes. Remove from heat and let stand for 2–3 hours. Drain well. Cover again with cold water to about ½ inch over the top of the beans. Bring to a boil, reduce heat, cover, and let simmer for about 2½ hours or until the beans are soft.

Thoroughly mix beans with remaining ingredients. Place in a shallow baking dish and bake, uncovered, at 325° F. for 2 to 3 hours or until the beans are rather dry, stirring every hour. Serve hot or cold, using ⅓ cup beans per serving.

	CAL	CHO (gm)	PRO (gm)	FAT (gm)	NA (mg)
Nutritive values per serving:	115	18	7	2	262

Food exchanges per serving: 1 bread, 1 lean meat
Low-sodium diets: Omit salt.

RED BEANS AND RICE

Yields 6 cups—12 servings

Judy Ballantine from Greensboro, North Carolina, loves this combination. It takes a lot of exhanges but she says it is worth it even though it takes most of the exchanges for a meal.

1 pound dry kidney beans
Water as necessary
1 cup chopped onions
¾ cup chopped fresh green peppers
1 cup finely chopped celery
4 ounces chopped center-cut ham with fat, skin, and bone removed
2 teaspoons salt
½ teaspoon cayenne pepper
¼ teaspoon black pepper
3 tablespoons thinly sliced green onion tops
1½ tablespoons parsley flakes
6 cups hot fluffy cooked rice
Fresh onion slices

Wash and sort beans. Add 2 quarts hot water. Cover and soak overnight. Drain well. Discard the liquid and add cold water to cover the beans to about ½ inch over the top.

Add onions, peppers, celery, ham, salt, cayenne, and black pepper to beans. Bring to a boil. Reduce heat, cover, and simmer 2½ hours, stirring occasionally. Add onion tops and parsley to beans. Simmer uncovered about 30 minutes, stirring occasionally.

Serve ½ cup of the hot beans over ½ cup of the rice per serving. Garnish the beans with a few onion slices, if desired.

Nutritive values per serving including rice:	CAL	CHO (gm)	PRO (gm)	FAT (gm)	NA (mg)
	244	43	14	3	381

Food exchanges per serving: 2 bread, 1 milk
Low-sodium diets: Omit salt.

CREAMY BROWN RICE

Yields 3 cups—9 servings

I never really liked brown rice until Dr. Karen Kuenzel of the Rice Research and Extension Center at the University of Arkansas told me that I wasn't using enough liquid and I wasn't cooking it long enough. She gave me these proportions to use and now I like it very much and use it more often. Dr. Kuenzel is the daughter of Zella Kuenzel, a friend of mine who is a dietitian in Guttenberg, Iowa, a town on the Mississippi near us. Dr. Kuenzel was in Guttenberg so I asked Zella if she would help me with my difficulties with brown rice—and she helped me a lot!

1 cup brown rice
2½ cups boiling water
½ teaspoon salt

Place rice, water, and salt in a Crockpot. Turn on high and cook for about 2 hours or until soft and creamy. Serve hot using ⅓ cup per serving.
Note: If you like brown rice more firm, use less liquid. It can also be cooked in a saucepan over low heat for about 50–60 minutes if you don't like to use the Crockpot. Remove the lid and fluff the rice with a fork, cover with a napkin or terry cloth dish towel, and let set 5–10 minutes to fluff before it is served, using ⅓ cup per serving.

Nutritive values per serving:	CAL	CHO (gm)	PRO (gm)	FAT (gm)	NA (mg)
	74	16	2	negl.	239
Food exchanges per serving:	1 bread				
Low-sodium diets:	Omit salt.				

MEDIUM WHITE SAUCE

Yields 1 cup—4 servings

2 tablespoons all-purpose flour
¼ cup instant dry milk
½ teaspoon salt
¹⁄₁₆ teaspoon white pepper (optional)
1 tablespoon vegetable oil
1 cup cold water

Stir together flour, milk, salt, and pepper until blended. Set aside for later use. Place oil in a small saucepan. Add the flour mixture and cook and stir over moderate heat until smooth but not browned. Remove from heat.

Add 1 cup water to flour mixture. Return to heat and cook and stir over medium heat until sauce is thickened and smooth. (1 cup fat-free chicken broth may be substituted for the cold water, if desired, to make a Velouté sauce with no change in food exchanges. However, the sodium will be increased to 546 mg per serving.) Use for creamed vegetables or meats using ¼ cup per serving.

Nutritive values per serving:

	CAL	CHO (gm)	PRO (gm)	FAT (gm)	NA (mg)
	68	5	2	5	524

Food exchanges per serving: ½ milk, 1 fat
Low-sodium diets: Omit salt.

BLINTZES

Yields 18 blintzes—6 servings

This recipe is from Anita Kane of Shorewood, Wisconsin. Anita serves them with unsweetened applesauce or other fruit. I like them with Cinnamon Shake or Apple Butter (see index).

FILLING
1 pound well-drained low-fat cottage cheese
¼ cup liquid egg substitute
2 teaspoons sugar

PANCAKE
¾ cup liquid egg substitute
1 cup water
¾ cup all-purpose flour
2 tablespoons vegetable oil
Margarine or oil as necessary

Mix cottage cheese, ¼ cup egg substitute, and sugar together lightly and refrigerate until needed.

Beat together ¾ cup egg substitute, 1 cup water, flour, and 2 tablespoons oil until smooth.

Heat a little margarine or oil in a 6-inch frying pan (I like oil best). Use a shallow frying pan as you would for frying crepes. Pour about 2 tablespoons batter into the frying pan, tilting the pan so that the batter coats as much of the pan surface as possible. It should make a very thin pancake. Cook over medium heat 1 to 2 minutes or until the bottom of the pancake is lightly browned and the sides are curled up. Carefully turn the pancake out onto a clean dish towel. The pancakes can be stacked like shingles.

When all of the pancakes are cooked, spread about a tablespoon of filling in the center of each pancake. Fold in both sides and then the ends so that you have a neat little package. Place the blintzes seam side down in a baking dish that has been greased with margarine. Brush lightly with melted margarine and bake at 375° F. for 30–40 minutes or until browned and puffy. Serve hot with fruit, Apple Butter, or Cinnamon Shake (see index), using 3 blintzes per serving.

These freeze very well. I put them individually on a cookie sheet until they are frozen and then I keep them in a bag in the freezer until I need them. I grease a baking dish well with margarine and let them defrost before I bake them.

Nutritive values per serving without fat used for frying and to top blintzes when they are baked:	CAL	CHO (gm)	PRO (gm)	FAT (gm)	NA (mg)
	180	16	17	5	254

Food exchanges per serving: 1 bread, 2 lean meat
Low-sodium diets: Use salt-free margarine.

MOCK SOUR CREAM

Yields 2 cups—8 servings

This recipe from Esther Smith, a home economist from near Wadena, is great on baked potatoes. I also like to add some garlic powder to it and use it as a dip or for salad dressing.

1½ cups well-drained cottage cheese, preferably large curd
2 tablespoons dry buttermilk
½ cup skim milk
1 tablespoon lemon juice
½ teaspoon salt

Place all ingredients in bowl of food processor and process until thick and smooth. Refrigerate until needed using ¼ cup per serving.

Nutritive values per serving:	CAL	CHO (gm)	PRO (gm)	FAT (gm)	NA (mg)
	46	3	8	negl.	260

Food exchanges per serving: 1 lean meat, ¼ milk
Low-sodium diets: Omit salt.

STEWED CRANBERRIES

Yields 3 cups—6 servings

I like cranberries very much and like to keep a supply of them in the freezer. I always buy several packages when they first come to our stores in the fall and stew them, or freeze them whole, to have all winter.

1 pound fresh cranberries
1 cup water
Sugar substitute equal to ½ cup sugar

Wash cranberries well under running water. Pick them over and discard any imperfect berries. Place cranberries and water in a small saucepan. Simmer about 5 minutes or until the cranberries have burst.

Remove from heat. Add sugar substitute, mix lightly, and cool to room temperature. Taste for flavor and add more sugar substitute, if desired. Refrigerate until used, using ½ cup per serving.

Nutritive values per serving:	CAL	CHO (gm)	PRO (gm)	FAT (gm)	NA (mg)
	33	8	negl.	negl.	negl.
Food exchanges per serving:	1 vegetable (2 tablespoons may be considered free)				
Low-sodium diets:	May be used as written.				

12
SALADS AND SALAD DRESSINGS

Salads are an important part of a diabetic diet. A chef's salad is easy to order when you are eating out, and a bowl of lettuce added to your lunch or dinner makes you feel as though you have dined well—which you have. Salads offer bulk, fiber, vitamins and minerals, satisfaction, and good taste, all of which are very important. However, you need to be careful even when ordering or making a salad because some salads can hide a lot of cholesterol and carbohydrate, and the most innocent-looking fruit salad can hide a lot of fat in the dressing. So always analyze a salad (quietly to yourself, of course) before you eat it.

Some salad ingredients are so low in calories that you can eat up to a cup of them without counting them, so I always try to include them in salads whenever possible. They include chinese cabbage, cucumbers, endive, escarole, lettuce, parsley, dill pickles, radishes, and watercress.

A good tossed salad begins with clean, crisp greens. They lose texture and nutrients even when properly refrigerated so it is best to be careful when you are preparing them. They are also fragile and must be stored carefully. It is a good idea not to wash them until shortly before they are used. Everyone has different ideas about how to keep greens fresh. I like to clean them and remove as much of the water as possible, and then store them in a plastic container in the refrigerator until I need them. Some cooks like to wash them and wrap them in a damp towel and refrigerate them until used. If they are wilted you can sometimes bring them back to a manageable state by soaking them in cold water for a short time and then drying them before they are used. Remember, you shouldn't add the dressing until just before the salad is served because the dressing will wilt the greens.

Hard-cooked egg yolks should not be used in a salad on a low-cholesterol diabetic diet because of the cholesterol in the egg yolks. If you want chopped whole eggs in your salad, you can cook liquid egg substitute in the microwave oven or the top of a double boiler, let it return to room temperature, and then chop it into cubes for use in salads. I generally just hard-cook the eggs, discard the egg yolks, and chop the whites for salad. You can use the egg yolks to garnish the salad, and anyone who doesn't need to watch their cholesterol intake can eat them. Don't feel guilty if you throw away the yolks. Just tell yourself you are discarding cholesterol and it gets easier every time you do it.

There are some good low-calorie salad dressings on the market that are suitable for a low-cholesterol diabetic recipe. However, they hardly ever contain vegetable oil because of the calories, and you do need some polyunsaturated vegetable oils in your diet. Anyone on a low-cholesterol diabetic diet has a hard time balancing the amount of vegetable oil needed for his low-cholesterol diet with the number of fat exchanges on his diabetic diet. I suggest that you talk to your doctor about it and see which is the most important—getting the polyunsaturated vegetable oil or restricting your fat intake.

Sour cream is also a no-no on a low-cholesterol diet and a lot of very good dressings contain sour cream. You can generally substitute low-fat yogurt for sour cream in most recipes with good results. Again, it is a good idea to read the list of ingredients on the container before you buy salad dressing to be sure they don't contain anything that shouldn't be used on a low-cholesterol diet—as well as honey, or sugar, or other things that shouldn't be used on a diabetic diet. I'm happy to say that Miracle Whip, made by Kraft, is satisfactory on a low-cholesterol diet—it is very low in cholesterol and is low enough in carbohydrate that it can also be used on a diabetic diet (within reason, of course). If you are in doubt about your favorite dressing, read the label; you may be happily surprised.

Fruits and vegetables—except for coconut and coconut oil and palm oil—do not have any cholesterol. You are free to use any fruits and vegetables in a salad that will fit into your diabetic diet pattern. I haven't used any avocados because they are so high in fat exchanges that they are hard to fit into a diabetic diet pattern. However, if you like them well enough that you are willing to use your fat exchanges for them, feel perfectly free to use them; they are a good source of fiber, which is a plus. I also have not used grapefruit or oranges because I feel that most diabetics use them so often and are so used to eating them that I should concentrate on salads that might be a little different. Grapefruit sections or orange sections on a lettuce leaf is a perfect salad for both the low-cholesterol and diabetic diets.

Equal (aspartame) sugar substitute has been used a great deal in this chapter because I like to use it whenever possible, but feel free to use your own favorite sugar substitute. Each packet of Equal is equal to 2 teaspoons sugar—use your own favorite sugar substitute accordingly.

BASIC SALAD GELATIN

Yields about 2 cups—4 servings

This gelatin base is free and doesn't need to be counted. However, you will need to count any other ingredients that you add to the gelatin unless they, too, are free.

1¾ cups water
1 ¼-ounce packet Knox Unflavored Gelatine
2 tablespoons lemon juice or white vinegar
Sugar substitute equal to 2 tablespoons sugar

Place 1 cup water in pan. Sprinkle gelatin over it and let set for 5 minutes. Heat and stir over low heat until clear and gelatin is dissolved. Remove from heat.

Add remaining ¾ cup water, lemon juice, and sweetener to gelatin mixture. Stir to dissolve sugar substitute, if necessary. Pour into mold or dish and refrigerate until firm. Serve about ½ cup per serving. (Up to 1½ cups vegetables or fruit may be added to the gelatin. First chill the gelatin until it is the consistency of unbeaten egg whites. Then fold in vegetables and pour into mold or bowl. Chill until firm.)

Nutritive values per serving: May be used as desired without adding any
                                   nutritive value.
Food exchanges per serving: None
Low-sodium diets: May be used as written.

FRUIT-FLAVORED GELATIN

Yields 2 cups—4 servings

You can use any flavor unsweetened drink mix with this recipe, but we prefer strawberry or cherry. Of course, you will have to calculate any fruit or other ingredients you add to the gelatin. If you add 1 cup drained, unsweetened fruit to the gelatin, each serving will be ½ fruit exchange.

2 cups water
1 ¼-ounce packet Knox Unflavored Gelatine
1 .20-ounce packet Wyler's unsweetened flavored soft drink mix or Kool-Ald unsweetened soft drink mix
8 1-gram packets Equal (aspartame) sugar substitute

Sprinkle gelatin over water. Heat over low heat or in the microwave oven until water is hot and gelatin is dissolved. Add drink mix and sweetener to hot gelatin mixture and stir until dissolved. Pour into mold or dish and refrigerate until firm. Serve ½ cup per serving.

Nutritive values per serving:	CAL	CHO (gm)	PRO (gm)	FAT (gm)	NA (mg)
	8	2	negl.	negl.	negl.

Food exchanges per serving: 1 serving may be considered free
Low-sodium diets: May be used as written.

APPLE SALAD

Yields 1 9-inch square pan—12 servings

This recipe is from Kay Knochel of Phoenix, Arizona. It is a typically Midwestern recipe which she gave me when we were roommates in Chicago.

Diabetic lemon gelatin to prepare 2 cups gelatin
1¾ cups water
½ cup low-fat cottage cheese
2 small (4 to the pound) tart apples
½ cup chopped nuts

Prepare gelatin according to directions, using 1¾ cups water instead of 2 cups. Refrigerate until it begins to thicken. Drain cottage cheese well and mash with the back of a large spoon. Fold into slightly thickened gelatin. Wash and core apples but do not peel them. Cut into small pieces and stir into the gelatin.

Stir nuts into gelatin and pour into a 9-inch square pan that has been rinsed with cold water. Chill until firm. Cut 3 × 4 into 12 equal portions. Serve 1 portion on a lettuce leaf per serving. The salad may be garnished with 1 tablespoon Kay's Cooked Dressing (see index) without adding any exchanges, if desired.

Nutritive values per serving:	CAL	CHO (gm)	PRO (gm)	FAT (gm)	NA (mg)
	51	4	2	3	30

Food exchanges per serving: 1 vegetable, ½ fat
Low-sodium diets: May be used as written. Use the low-sodium variation if Kay's Cooked Dressing is used.

MOLDED SPICY APRICOT SALAD

Yields 1 8-inch square—6 servings

This salad is excellent for buffets. It is colorful, and the surprising, spicy taste is a good accent to cold roast meats, chicken, and turkey.

1 16-ounce can apricot halves in light syrup
¼ cup white vinegar
2 tablespoons sugar
1 stick cinnamon
4 whole cloves
Water
1 .3-ounce package apricot or peach sugar-free gelatin
3 1-gram packets Equal (aspartame) sugar substitute

Drain apricots well and reserve liquid. Refrigerate apricots. Combine apricot juice, vinegar, sugar, cinnamon, and cloves. Add enough water to yield 2 cups liquid. Pour into a saucepan, cover, and simmer for 10 minutes. Immediately strain spices from liquid and dissolve gelatin in liquid while still hot. Add enough cold water to total 2 cups, if necessary. Stir Equal into gelatin mixture and mix lightly. Cool until syrupy, add apricots, mix lightly, and pour into 8-inch-square glass dish and refrigerate until set. Cut into 6 equal portions, using 1 portion per serving. (The gelatin can also be molded and ½ cup of the salad used per serving.)

Nutritive values per serving:	CAL	CHO (gm)	PRO (gm)	FAT (gm)	NA (mg)
	60	14	1	0	3

Food exchanges per serving: 1 fruit
Low-sodium diets: May be used as written.

NECTARINE SALAD

Yields 3 cups—6 servings

If nectarines aren't available, you can use ½ cup well-drained, sliced, juice-packed peaches instead.

¼ cup Miracle Whip salad dressing
¼ cup 2% milk
1 1-gram packet Equal (aspartame) sugar substitute
2 cups diced crisp, fresh apples (about 2 medium-size)
1 cup sliced, washed but not peeled, fresh nectarine (about 1 medium)
1 cup diced celery

Place Miracle Whip, milk, and Equal in a bowl and mix until smooth. Let sit at room temperature for 15 minutes to thicken. Add apples, nectarine, and celery. Mix lightly and refrigerate. Serve cold, using ½ cup per serving.

Nutritive values per serving:	CAL	CHO (gm)	PRO (gm)	FAT (gm)	NA (mg)
	107	11	1	5	102

Food exchanges per serving: ⅔ fruit, 1 fat
Low-sodium diets: May be used as written.

CRANBERRY GELATIN SALAD

Yields 1 9-inch square mold—12 servings

Diabetic strawberry gelatin to yield 4 cups gelatin
2 cups water
1¼ cups cooked cranberries, unsweetened
½ cup finely chopped celery
¼ cup Kay's Cooked Dressing (see index)
¼ cup chopped nuts
Sugar substitute

Prepare gelatin as directed on the package using only 1¾ cups water. Cool for 5 minutes. Add cranberries, celery, dressing, and nuts to gelatin mixture. Mix lightly.

Add sweetener to salad to taste. Pour salad into a 9-inch square glass pan. Refrigerate until firm. Cut 3 × 4 into 12 equal portions. Serve 1 square on a lettuce leaf per serving. The salad may be garnished with 1 teaspoon Kay's Cooked Dressing without changing the exchange values.

Nutritive values per serving:	CAL	CHO (gm)	PRO (gm)	FAT (gm)	NA (mg)
	25	2	1	1	21

Food exchanges per serving: One serving may be considered free
Low-sodium diets: May be used as written. Use low-sodium variation of salad dressing.

BROCCOLI SALAD

Yields 4½ cups—9 servings

This recipe is based on one from Esther Smith. Esther is a home economist who lives out in the country near Wadena. She is in charge of the school lunch program at our local school and plays the organ at our church. This tremendously talented person is also a marvelous seamstress and a wonderful program chairman for our Federated Club here in Wadena—the sort of person that every small town needs.

2 cups sliced fresh cauliflower
2 cups sliced fresh broccoli
⅓ cup sliced Bermuda onion
1 teaspoon garlic salt
1 cup sliced fresh mushrooms
3 tablespoons Miracle Whip salad dressing
1 tablespoon milk

Clean the cauliflower, broccoli, and onion and slice them evenly. I like to trim the skin from the stalks of the broccoli and use the stalks, saving the flowerets for a vegetable. However, I do use the cauliflower flowerets, slicing them lengthwise—they look so pretty together that way.

Sprinkle the garlic salt over the vegetables. Toss them lightly and place them in a covered container in the refrigerator overnight.

Drain broccoli mixture well and add sliced mushrooms. Thoroughly mix together salad dressing and milk and pour over the vegetables. Mix lightly and serve ½ cup per serving.

Nutritive values per serving:

	CAL	CHO (gm)	PRO (gm)	FAT (gm)	NA (mg)
	44	4	2	1	270

Food exchanges per serving: 1 vegetable
Low-sodium diets: Run a little cold water over the broccoli mixture after you drain off the salt water.

SPECIAL BROCCOLI SALAD

Yields 4⅔ cups—7 servings

This is another broccoli salad from Esther Smith. We both like broccoli, so we are always looking for new and different broccoli recipes for our recipe files.

¼ cup Miracle Whip salad dressing
¼ cup skim milk
1 tablespoon white vinegar
3 1-gram packets Equal (aspartame) sugar substitute
¼ teaspoon salt
1 quart fresh broccoli flowerlets and sliced, peeled stems
2 tablespoons raisins
2 tablespoons salted sunflower kernels
½ cup chopped onions

Combine Miracle Whip and milk in a mixing bowl and stir until smooth. Add vinegar, sugar substitute, and salt and mix well. Let sit at room temperature for 15–30 minutes.

Prepare broccoli and set aside. Add raisins, sunflower kernels, and onions to Miracle Whip mixture. Mix lightly, pour over broccoli, mix lightly again, and refrigerate 2–8 hours before serving. Serve chilled using ⅔ cup salad per serving.

Nutritive values per serving:	CAL	CHO (gm)	PRO (gm)	FAT (gm)	NA (mg)
	91	9	3	2	158

Food exchanges per serving: 2 vegetable
Low-sodium diets: Omit salt. Use unsalted sunflower kernels.

MARINATED BROCCOLI AND MUSHROOMS

Yields 6 cups—8 servings

My godchild, Vicki Glastetter, from Redlands, California, shared this recipe with me. She arranges the broccoli flowerlets around the edge of the platter and piles the mushrooms in the center for an appetizer that she says she and her friends enjoy. I use it as a salad because it is so pretty and tastes so good. She uses ½ teaspoon pepper, but I use only ⅛ teaspoon pepper. Our taste buds aren't used to the hot Southwestern food that she and her friends enjoy.

1½ pounds fresh broccoli
8 ounces fresh mushrooms
½ cup tarragon vinegar
1 tablespoon chopped parsley
⅛–½ teaspoon pepper
½ teaspoon salt
1 tablespoon lemon juice
¼ cup vegetable oil
1 tablespoon sugar
2 large cloves garlic

Wash broccoli and cut into bite-size pieces. Place in a plastic or stainless-steel refrigerator container that has a tight cover. Wash or wipe off mushrooms, thinly slice them, and place on top of broccoli.

In a separate bowl, combine vinegar, parsley, pepper, salt, lemon juice, oil, and sugar. Mash or chop garlic very fine and add to dressing. Mix well and pour over vegetables. Cover container tightly and refrigerate, turning container over several times a day, for 2 or 3 days. Drain well and serve, using ¾ cup per serving.

	CAL	CHO (gm)	PRO (gm)	FAT (gm)	NA (mg)
Nutritive values per serving:	56	5	2	4	82

Food exchanges per serving: 1 vegetable, 1 fat
Low-sodium diets: Omit salt.

CARROT AND PINEAPPLE SALAD

Yields about 2 cups—4 servings

This is the salad I make for my sister Shirley when she is here because she likes it so well.

2 cups shredded carrots
½ cup canned unsweetened crushed pineapple with juice
1 tablespoon raisins
¼ cup Kay's Cooked Dressing (see index)
1 tablespoon lemon juice
⅛ teaspoon salt
1 1-gram packet Equal (aspartame) sugar substitute

Place carrots, pineapple, and raisins in small mixing bowl.

Stir together dressing, lemon juice, salt, and sweetener to blend and add to carrot mixture. Toss lightly to coat carrot mixture with dressing and refrigerate until served. Serve ¼ of the salad (about ½ cup) for each serving.

Nutritive values per serving:	CAL	CHO (gm)	PRO (gm)	FAT (gm)	NA (mg)
	51	10	1	1	134

Food exchanges per serving: ⅔ fruit
Low-sodium diets: Omit salt. Use low-sodium variation of salad dressing.

CHEF'S SALAD

Yields 1 salad—1 serving

I'm sure I don't need to tell you about chef's salad. We so often order them in restaurants since it is the easiest thing to order to count our exchanges and not go over. They come in all varieties and forms, but this version is my favorite for preparing at home.

1 cup chopped or shredded fresh crisp lettuce
¼ medium-size fresh, washed, cored, and sliced or diced tomato
¼ cup chopped celery
¼ cup chopped onions
½ cup sliced fresh cauliflower
1 ounce (about 3 tablespoons) diced or chopped cooked chicken with
 all visible fat removed
1 ounce (about 3 tablespoons) diced or chopped lean ham with all
 visible fat removed
¼ cup Garlic Dressing (see index)

Place lettuce evenly in the bottom of a shallow salad bowl. (I often use a shallow soup bowl for my salad.) Sprinkle tomato, celery, onions, and cauliflower evenly over chopped lettuce.

Sprinkle chicken and ham evenly over chopped vegetables. (You can use sliced chicken and ham, if desired, and cut the slices into strips instead of dicing them.) Pour dressing evenly over salad, or keep on the side and use as needed. Serve salad chilled. Serve all of the salad for 1 serving.

Nutritive values per serving:

CAL	CHO (gm)	PRO (gm)	FAT (gm)	NA (mg)
250	15	22	5	132

Food exchanges per serving: 3 vegetable, 2 lean meat
Low-sodium diets: Use 2 ounces chicken instead of 1 ounce chicken and 1 ounce ham, unless the ham is mild and not very salty. Use the low-sodium variation of the salad dressing.

COLESLAW

Yields about 1½ quarts—12 servings

Coleslaw has always been a favorite of ours so I generally make a pretty good-sized batch of it. You can make it the day before a party or a picnic because it is even better the second day.

1½ pounds (about 3 quarts) cleaned, cored, and shredded cabbage
1½ cups shredded carrots
¼ cup chopped fresh green peppers
¼ cup finely chopped onions
2 tablespoons chopped parsley
¾ cup Kay's Cooked Dressing (see index)
¼ cup vinegar
1 tablespoon celery seed
2 teaspoons salt
Sugar substitute equal to ⅓ cup sugar

Place cabbage in the bottom of a big mixing bowl. Add remaining vegetables and toss lightly.

Mix together dressing, vinegar, celery seed, salt, and sweetener until smooth and pour over the vegetables. Mix lightly, cover, and refrigerate at least 2 hours. Toss salad and dressing again just before it is served. Drain excess liquid from the salad and allow ½ cup salad per serving.

Nutritional values per serving:

CAL	CHO (gm)	PRO (gm)	FAT (gm)	NA (mg)
36	6	1	1	231

Food exchanges per serving: 1 vegetable
Low-sodium diets: Omit salt. Use low-sodium variation of salad dressing.

TRADITIONAL CABBAGE SALAD

Yields 4 cups—6 servings

This recipe is from M. J. Smith, a registered dietitian from Guttenberg, Iowa, a lovely little town on the Mississippi. She has been doing wonderful recipes with lower calorie counts for traditional foods.

1½ teaspoons salad mustard
Dry sugar substitute equal to ¼ cup sugar
1 tablespoon vegetable oil
¼ teaspoon salt
¼ teaspoon celery seed
2 tablespoons white vinegar
3 cups shredded cabbage
1½ cups shredded carrot
¼ cup shredded onions
½ cup chopped fresh green peppers

Combine mustard, sugar substitute, oil, salt, celery seed, and vinegar and set aside.

Place cabbage, carrots, onions, and green peppers in a mixing bowl. Shake dressing well and pour over vegetables. Mix lightly and refrigerate. Serve cold using ⅔ cup per serving.

Nutritive values per serving:	CAL	CHO (gm)	PRO (gm)	FAT (gm)	NA (mg)
	55	6	1	3	111

Food exchanges per serving: 1 vegetable, ½ fat
Low-sodium diets: Omit salt.

TONY'S SNAPPY COLESLAW

Yields 1 quart—8 servings

Nellie Yurkovich gave me this recipe, which her late husband, Tony, developed one day when he couldn't find any sweet green peppers. It was such a success that he continued to make it. Tony was an excellent cook and did a lot of cooking before and after they were married.

2 quarts shredded cabbage
½ cup shredded carrots
½ cup shredded red onions
½ cup finely chopped jalapeño peppers
½ cup vegetable oil
¼ cup white vinegar
1 tablespoon white sugar
2 teaspoons salt
½ teaspoon celery seed
¼ teaspoon black pepper

Place cabbage, carrots, onions, and jalapeño peppers in a bowl and toss lightly to mix well. In a separate bowl, stir together oil, vinegar, sugar, salt, celery seed, and black pepper to mix well. Add to vegetables and toss again. Cover and refrigerate for 3 hours before serving. Drain well and serve, using ½ cup per serving.

Nutritive values per serving:

	CAL	CHO (gm)	PRO (gm)	FAT (gm)	NA (mg)
	61	7	1	4	545

Food exchanges per serving: 1 vegetable, 1 fat

Low-sodium diets: Before you combine vegetables, sprinkle 2 teaspoons salt over cabbage and let sit for 1 hour. Rinse cabbage and then proceed with the rest of the recipe.

CUCUMBER SALAD

Yields about 2 cups—3 servings

Frances Sonitzky who gave me this recipe says it is a basic Hungarian recipe. You can add a little more or less onion, make it a little sweeter or add a whisper of white pepper according to your tastes.

2 small cucumbers 6–7 inches long
¾ teaspoon salt
2 tablespoons finely chopped onions
2 tablespoons white vinegar
2 tablespoons evaporated skim milk
2 1-gram packets Equal (aspartame) sugar substitute
Paprika

Slice cucumbers as thin as possible. Sprinkle with salt and let set at room temperature for 1–2 hours. Drain well and with your hands, squeeze as much juice as possible out of the cucumbers.

Mix onions, vinegar, milk, and sweetener together lightly. Add cucumbers and mix lightly. Refrigerate until ready to serve, using about ⅔ cup (⅓ of the finished recipe) per serving. Sprinkle each portion with paprika just before it is served.

Nutritive values per serving:	CAL	CHO (gm)	PRO (gm)	FAT (gm)	NA (mg)
	22	5	1	negl.	303

Food exchanges per serving: 1 vegetable

Low-sodium diets: Press as much of the juice out of the cucumbers as possible to eliminate as much of the salt as possible.

CUCUMBER AND LETTUCE SALAD

Yields about 6 cups—6 servings

This salad is light with a delicate flavor, a good accompaniment to a strongly flavored casserole.

1 small cucumber 6 to 7 inches long
½ teaspoon salt
1 tablespoon chopped parsley
2 tablespoons low-fat yogurt
¼ cup Kay's Cooked Dressing (see index)
2 tablespoons skim milk
6 cups fresh crisp lettuce

Peel cucumber and grate coarsely. Sprinkle with salt and refrigerate for ½ hour. Drain well, pressing as much juice as possible out of the cucumber. Combine parsley, yogurt, dressing, and milk with drained cucumbers and mix lightly.

Tear lettuce into bite-size pieces. Toss with cucumber mixture just before it is served, using about 1 cup lettuce per serving.

Nutritive values per serving:	CAL	CHO (gm)	PRO (gm)	FAT (gm)	NA (mg)
	25	3	1	1	124

Food exchanges per serving: ½ vegetable
Low-sodium diets: Press as much of the juice out of the cucumber as possible to eliminate as much of the salt as possible.

FARMER'S SALAD

Yields about 7½ cups—6 servings

I like to use warm, freshly cooked potatoes and green beans for this salad. They seem to absorb the flavor of the dressing better that way.

1 pound new potatoes
1 pound fresh green beans cut into 1-inch pieces
½ cup Vinaigrette Dressing (see index)
1½ cups (6 ounces) lean cubed cooked beef with all visible fat removed
Fresh crisp lettuce leaves as necessary
3 medium-size ripe red tomatoes
½ cup sliced sweet onions

Cook potatoes and green beans. Peel potatoes and slice them into about ¼-inch-thick slices. Place both potatoes and green beans in a mixing bowl. Pour dressing over potatoes and beans. Mix lightly, cover, and let sit about ½ hour at room temperature. Toss beef with marinated vegetables.

Line a round serving plate with lettuce leaves. Mound the vegetable and meat mixture in the center of the plate and surround it with tomato wedges and onions. Refrigerate if not served immediately (but it is better if served immediately). Serve ⅙ of the salad per serving.

Nutritive values per serving:	CAL	CHO (gm)	PRO (gm)	FAT (gm)	NA (mg)
	164	19	12	5	72

Food exchanges per serving: 1 bread, 1 vegetable, 1 lean meat
Low-sodium diets: Cook potatoes and beans without salt and use the low-sodium variation of the salad dressing.

FRIJOLE SALAD

Yields about 6 cups—12 servings

¾ cup rinsed and drained kidney beans
⅔ cup Spicy Tomato Dressing (see index)
4 cups shredded cabbage
½ cup thinly sliced sweet onions or green onions and tops
1 cup diced tomatoes (1 medium-size tomato)
½ cup peeled and thinly sliced cucumbers

Combine beans and dressing, mix lightly, cover, and refrigerate overnight.

Place cabbage in the bottom of a mixing bowl. Place beans with dressing, onions, tomatoes, and cucumbers over the cabbage. Toss lightly just before serving, using ½ cup per serving. Lettuce may be substituted for cabbage, if desired, without changing the exchange values.

Nutritive values per serving:	CAL	CHO (gm)	PRO (gm)	FAT (gm)	NA (mg)
	46	6	2	2	81

Food exchanges per serving: 1 vegetable
Low-sodium diets: Use beans without salt and use the low-sodium variation of the salad dressing.

GARDEN COTTAGE CHEESE SALAD

Yields 5 cups—10 servings

We use this at Health Care Manor Nursing Home in Hampton, Iowa, where I work as a dietary consultant. The employees like it as well as the residents do—it is popular with everyone at the home.

½ **cup thinly sliced radishes**
½ **cup finely chopped onions**
½ **cup finely chopped celery**
¼ **cup finely chopped fresh green peppers**
½ **cup thinly sliced cucumbers**
2 tablespoons Kay's Cooked Dressing (see index)
1 teaspoon salt
1½ **pounds low-fat cottage cheese**

Combine vegetables and toss lightly. Combine dressing and salt and stir into vegetables.

Drain cottage cheese well and add to vegetable mixture. Mix lightly and refrigerate until served. Drain off any liquid before it is served, using ½ cup of the mixture per serving. This should be prepared as close to serving time as possible.

You can use the same amounts of any other fresh raw vegetables you might prefer—such as chives, slivers of fresh cauliflower, or broccoli—without changing the exchange values.

Nutritive values per serving:	CAL	CHO (gm)	PRO (gm)	FAT (gm)	NA (mg)
	74	3	9	negl.	372

Food exchanges per serving: ¼ milk, 1 lean meat
Low-sodium diets: Omit salt. Use low-sodium variation of salad dressing.

INDIVIDUAL BEEF SALAD

Yields 1 salad—1 serving

I'm so fond of this salad and serve it so often when tomatoes are in season that I think Chuck gets tired of it—even though it was his mother's favorite salad and he taught me to make it when we were first married.

2 ounces (about ⅓ cup) chopped or cubed cooked lean beef with all visible fat removed
¼ cup chopped or sliced fresh sweet onions
¼ cup chopped fresh green peppers
2 tablespoons Spicy Tomato Dressing (see index)
1 large tomato
Lettuce leaf
½ teaspoon fresh parsley (optional)

Mix beef, onions, peppers, and dressing lightly in a small bowl. Cover and refrigerate 1–8 hours. Wash and core tomato. Cut into cubes or wedges. Add to marinated meat and dressing mixture and toss to coat tomato with dressing.

Line a salad bowl with lettuce. Mound salad in center of the lettuce. Sprinkle parsley on top of salad and serve immediately. Serve all of the salad for 1 serving.

Nutritive values per serving:	CAL	CHO (gm)	PRO (gm)	FAT (gm)	NA (mg)
	220	17	19	9	181

Food exchanges per serving: 2 lean meat, 1 vegetable, 1 milk
Low-sodium diets: Use the low-sodium variation of the salad
    dressing.

TACO SALAD

Yields 6 salads—6 servings

This recipe makes 6 salads, but I generally just make 2 at a time. I freeze the remaining meat in portions and then reheat them as needed in the microwave. This salad is best when the meal is slightly warm when added to the vegetables.

1 tablespoon vegetable oil
1 pound lean ground beef
2 quarts hot water
1 cup taco sauce
6 cups shredded lettuce
2 cups cubed fresh tomatoes
½ cup thinly sliced onions
½ cup diced fresh green peppers
¾ cup Spicy Tomato Dressing (see index)
6 large pitted black olives

Preheat a frying pan over medium heat for 1 minute. Swirl oil around bottom of pan, add meat, and cook and stir over medium heat until meat is well browned and separated.

Place meat in a colander and drain off as much fat as possible. Pour hot water over meat and then discard that liquid also. Rinse the frying pan with hot water, wipe it dry, and return meat to pan. Add taco sauce and cook, stirring frequently, over medium heat until sauce has evaporated. Remove from heat and keep warm until used or refrigerate until needed and then warm again.

Fill 6 salad bowls with 1 cup lettuce each, add ⅓ cup tomato cubes to each salad, and sprinkle each bowl with ⅙ of the onions, peppers, and Spicy Tomato Dressing. Slice each olive into thin slices and use as garnish for each salad. Serve as soon as possible using 1 salad per serving.

Nutritive values per serving:	CAL	CHO (gm)	PRO (gm)	FAT (gm)	NA (mg)
	213	20	17	8	844

Food exchanges per serving: 1 bread, 2 lean meat, 1 vegetable
Low-sodium diets: Use low-sodium taco sauce and the low-sodium version of the Spicy Tomato Dressing.

KIDNEY BEAN SALAD

Yields 3 cups—6 servings

The idea of adding apple to a bean or pea salad came from my cousin LaVerle Sniffin of Waterloo, Iowa. We all think it really improves the salad.

⅓ cup Kay's Cooked Dressing (see index)
1 tablespoon chopped pimiento
¼ cup finely chopped Mrs. Riley's Pickles (see index) or dill pickles
¼ cup finely chopped onions (optional)
1 cup thinly sliced celery
4 chopped hard-cooked large egg whites
1 cup washed and drained canned kidney beans
1 small (4 to a pound) tart apple

Place dressing, pimiento, pickle, onion, celery, and egg whites in a mixing bowl and mix lightly. (In order to get the hard-cooked egg whites, I hard-cook 4 eggs and then discard the yolks, or use them to garnish the salad of someone who doesn't need to worry about cholesterol.) Add kidney beans to dressing mix.

Wash, core, and slice apple. Add to salad. Toss lightly and serve ½ cup per serving.

Nutritive values per serving:

	CAL	CHO (gm)	PRO (gm)	FAT (gm)	NA (mg)
	97	15	7	1	272

Food exchanges per serving: 1 milk

Low-sodium diets: Use only 2 tablespoons chopped pickles and the low-sodium variation of the salad dressing.

MARINATED VEGETABLE SALAD

Yields 7 cups—9 servings

1 cup water
1 tablespoon cornstarch
1 tablespoon prepared mustard
¼ cup lemon juice
6 1-gram packets Equal (aspartame) sugar substitute
2 cups broccoli flowerets
2 cups cauliflower flowerets
1 cup cooked celery
¼ cup chopped fresh green peppers
¼ cup chopped onions
½ cup drained and chopped pimientos
½ cup cooked and drained red beans
9 lettuce leaves

Stir water and cornstarch together until smooth in a small saucepan. Add mustard and cook and stir over moderate heat until thickened. Continue to cook and stir for 2 minutes. Remove from heat. Cool to room temperature. Add lemon juice and sweetener to sauce. Mix lightly and set aside for later use.

Place broccoli and cauliflower in boiling salted water and cook exactly 6 minutes after the water has returned to a boil. Drain immediately and cool to room temperature. Place in the bottom of a refrigerator bowl. Add celery, peppers, onions, pimientos, and beans to broccoli and cauliflower. Pour reserved dressing over the vegetables and mix lightly. Refrigerate overnight or all day. Toss lightly again just before serving.

Line each salad bowl with a crisp lettuce leaf. Add ¾ cup marinated vegetables per serving and serve chilled.

Nutritive values per serving:	CAL	CHO (gm)	PRO (gm)	FAT (gm)	NA (mg)
	46	9	3	1	48

Food exchanges per serving: 1½ vegetable
Low-sodium diets: Cook vegetables in unsalted water. (The amount of salt added in cooking the vegetable is not counted in the total sodium.)

POTATO SALAD

Yields 4 cups—8 servings

I like to make this several hours before I want to use it so the flavors can develop as the salad marinates.

1 cup Kay's Cooked Dressing (see index)
1 teaspoon salad mustard
1 1-gram packet Equal (aspartame) sugar substitute
½ teaspoon salt
Whisper of white pepper
1 tablespoon chopped parsley
¼ cup chopped Mrs. Riley's Pickles (see index) or dill pickles
¼ cup finely chopped onions (optional)
¼ cup chopped pimientos
½ cup finely chopped celery
4 chopped hard-cooked egg whites
3 cups cooked, peeled, and diced potatoes

Place dressing, mustard, sweetener, salt, pepper, and parsley in mixing bowl and mix lightly. Add pickles, onion, pimiento, celery, and egg whites to dressing and mix lightly. (That's right, don't use the egg yolks. Hard-cook the eggs, separate the yolks and whites and add the whites to the salad. I use the yolks as a garnish, and those who can have the egg yolks add them to their salad.)

Add potatoes and toss lightly to coat the potatoes well. Refrigerate until needed, serving ½ cup per serving.

Nutritive values per serving:	CAL	CHO (gm)	PRO (gm)	FAT (gm)	NA (mg)
	89	14	4	2	357

Food exchanges per serving: 1 bread
Low-sodium diets: Omit salt. Use the low-sodium variation of the salad dressing and cook the potatoes without salt.

SAUERKRAUT SALAD

Yields 6 cups—12 servings

This recipe is based on one from my cousin Ruth Clapper of Clear Lake, Iowa. I rinse the sauerkraut to make it milder but you can use it without rinsing if you like a stronger flavor.

3½ cups (29-ounce can) sauerkraut
⅓ cup white vinegar
3 tablespoons vegetable oil
½ cup water
8 1-gram packets Equal (aspartame) sugar substitute
½ cup chopped fresh green peppers
½ cup chopped onions
½ cup chopped and drained canned pimientos
1 cup thinly sliced celery

Drain sauerkraut well. Rinse with cold water and set aside to drain for later use.

Combine vinegar, oil, and water in a small saucepan. Bring to a boil and remove from heat. Add sweetener to hot vinegar and mix lightly.

Place drained sauerkraut in mixing bowl. Add remaining vegetables and mix lightly. Pour hot liquid over vegetables and mix again. Place in container, cover tightly, and refrigerate at least overnight before it is served. Serve ½ cup per serving.

Nutritive values per serving:	CAL	CHO (gm)	PRO (gm)	FAT (gm)	NA (mg)
	54	6	1	4	526

Food exchanges per serving: 1 vegetable, 1 fat
Low-sodium diets: This recipe is not suitable.

SWEET COLESLAW

Yields 5 cups—10 servings

This recipe from Gena LeVan of Royalton, Illinois, keeps practically forever in the refrigerator. I like to make it ahead of time to take to pot luck dinners. It stays crisp and good and everyone seems to like it very well.

2¾ cups ice water
1½ tablespoons salt
1 quart shredded cabbage
½ cup shredded fresh green peppers
¾ cup vinegar
1½ teaspoons mustard seed
2 cups thinly sliced celery
7 1-gram packets Equal (aspartame) sugar substitute
½ cup chopped, canned, drained pimientos

Place 2 cups water and salt in bowl and stir to dissolve salt. Add cabbage and peppers to cold salt water. Mix well and let set ½–1 hour.

Place vinegar, ¾ cup water, and mustard seed in a small saucepan and bring to a boil. Remove from heat. Immediately add celery to hot vinegar mixture. Cover and let cool to room temperature. Drain well, reserving liquid. Add sweetener to cool vinegar liquid.

Drain cabbage mixture well. Combine cabbage mixture, pimientos, and celery and vinegar mixture. Mix well. Refrigerate until needed. Serve ½ cup per serving.

Nutritive values per serving:

CAL	CHO (gm)	PRO (gm)	FAT (gm)	NA (mg)
20	5	1	negl.	143

Food exchanges per serving: 1 vegetable
Low-sodium diets: Wash cabbage very well with running cold water after it has soaked in the salted ice water or use salt substitute for soaking cabbage.

THREE-BEAN SALAD

Yields 7 cups—14 servings

Dried beans are high in fiber and we should try to eat a lot of them. However, they are also high in carbohydrate, so I generally try to mix them with something else that isn't all that high in carbohydrate. This salad recipe comes from my very good neighbor, Jan Franks, who is a nurse and is very much interested in good nutrition for herself and her family.

2 cups (16-ounce can) cooked, drained yellow wax beans cut into 1-inch lengths
2 cups (16-ounce can) cooked, drained green string beans cut into 1-inch lengths
½ cup washed and drained cooked kidney beans
1 cup thinly sliced onions
1 cup coarsely chopped fresh green peppers
1 cup thinly sliced celery
1 cup vinegar
⅛ teaspoon salt
Sugar substitute equal to ½ cup sugar

Place beans, onions, peppers, and celery in mixing bowl. Mix together vinegar, salt, and sweetener and pour over vegetables. Mix lightly, cover, and refrigerate at least overnight before serving ½ cup per serving.

Nutritive values per serving:	CAL	CHO (gm)	PRO (gm)	FAT (gm)	NA (mg)
	31	7	2	negl.	194

Food exchanges per serving: 1 vegetable
Low-sodium diets: Omit salt. Use vegetables canned without salt or an equal amount of fresh or frozen vegetables cooked without salt.

WALNUT WILD RICE

Yields 5 cups—10 servings

This recipe from Dr. Crockett's niece, Jacalyn Hill of Rancho Palos Verde, California, may be used as a salad or a potato substitute. We like it as a potato substitute with chicken, in which case I serve it lukewarm without chilling it.

1 6-ounce package Uncle Ben's long-grain and wild rice
1 cup thinly sliced celery
2 tablespoons chopped celery leaves
1 cup shredded carrots
4 tablespoons vegetable oil, divided
¼ cup chopped English walnuts
2 tablespoons red wine vinegar
1 1-gram packet Equal (aspartame) sugar substitute
1 teaspoon salt

Prepare rice according to the directions on the package, omitting the butter. Transfer rice to a large bowl and cool to room temperature. Stir celery, celery leaves, and carrots into cooked rice.

Place 2 tablespoons oil in a small frying pan. Add walnuts and cook and stir over medium heat until walnuts are golden and toasted. Remove from heat. Combine 2 tablespoons oil, vinegar, sweetener, and salt. Add to walnuts; mix lightly and pour over rice mixture. Toss lightly to blend well. Cover and chill well. Serve as a potato substitute or salad using ½ cup per serving.

Nutritive values per serving:

CAL	CHO (gm)	PRO (gm)	FAT (gm)	NA (mg)
136	15	10	7	237

Food exchanges per serving: 1 bread, 1 fat
Low-sodium diets: Omit salt.

ZUCCHINI SALAD

Yields about 2 quarts—16 servings

This recipe from Thelma VanLaningham of Independence, Iowa, is a delicious way to use those zucchini that grow so profusely in all our gardens.

²/₃ **cup cider vinegar**
2 tablespoons wine vinegar
2 tablespoons vegetable oil
½ **teaspoon pepper**
1 teaspoon salt
Liquid sugar substitute equal to ½ cup sugar
½ **cup diced onions**
½ **cup diced celery**
½ **cup diced fresh green peppers**
6 medium (about 6 to 7 inches) zucchini, washed and sliced

Combine vinegars, oil, pepper, salt, and sweetener and set aside for later use. Place vegetables in a mixing bowl and toss lightly. Add dressing and toss again. Cover and allow to marinate in the refrigerator at least 4 hours or overnight before it is served, using ½ cup per serving.

Nutritional values per serving:	CAL	CHO (gm)	PRO (gm)	FAT (gm)	NA (mg)
	31	4	1	2	143

Food exchanges per serving: 1 vegetable
Low-sodium diets: Omit salt.

KAY'S COOKED DRESSING

Yields 1¾ cups—14 servings

This creamy cooked dressing is from Kay Knochel of Phoenix, Arizona. Kay gave it to me when we were roommates in Chicago. She has always been an excellent cook and I still have several of her very good recipes in my personal file.

2 tablespoons cornstarch
2 teaspoons dry mustard
1 cup water
½ cup liquid egg substitute
¼ teaspoon salt
2 tablespoons margarine
½ cup white wine vinegar
6 1-gram packets Equal (aspartame) sugar substitute

Stir cornstarch, mustard, and water together until smooth in a 2-quart heavy saucepan. Add egg substitute, salt, and margarine to liquid in saucepan and mix well. Cook, stirring constantly, over low heat until thickened and smooth. Continue to simmer for 1 more minute, stirring constantly. Remove from heat.

Add vinegar and sweetener to dressing and mix well. Cover and refrigerate until used. Serve 2 tablespoons per serving.

Nutritive values per serving:

CAL	CHO (gm)	PRO (gm)	FAT (gm)	NA (mg)
27	2	1	2	80

Food exchanges per serving: Up to 2 tablespoons may be considered free
Low-sodium diets: Omit salt. Use salt-free margarine.

CREAMY GARLIC DRESSING

Yields 1 cup—8 servings

You can vary the amount of garlic powder used according to how much you like the taste of garlic. This is rather mild.

½ **cup Kay's Cooked Dressing (see index)**
½ **cup plain low-fat yogurt**
2 **tablespoons skim milk**
½ **teaspoon garlic powder**

Place all ingredients in a bowl and mix with a fork until smooth. Refrigerate in a covered container until served. Use 2 tablespoons per serving.

Nutritive values per serving:	CAL	CHO (gm)	PRO (gm)	FAT (gm)	NA (mg)
	20	2	1	1	14

Food exchanges per serving: 2 tablespoons may be considered free
Low-sodium diets: Use low-sodium variation of Kay's Cooked Dressing.

FRENCH DRESSING

Yields 2¼ cups—18 servings

1 cup vinegar
1 cup water
¼ cup vegetable oil
1 tablespoon paprika
1 teaspoon Worcestershire sauce
1 teaspoon A-1 sauce
½ teaspoon celery seed
1 teaspoon onion powder

Place all ingredients in a bowl and beat with a beater for ½ minute. Pour into a container, cover, and refrigerate until used. Bring back to room temperature and shake well before using. Allow 2 tablespoons per serving.

Nutritive values per serving:	CAL	CHO (gm)	PRO (gm)	FAT (gm)	NA (mg)
	31	1	negl.	3	4

Food exchanges per serving: ½ fat
Low-sodium diets: May be used as written.

SPICY TOMATO DRESSING

Yields 1½ cups—12 servings

This recipe is based on one from Anita Kane of Shorewood, Wisconsin. It is excellent on vegetables or lettuce and keeps well. If I intend to keep it more than a few days, however, I strain it to take out the dill weed and the onion.

1 cup (8 ounces) canned tomato sauce
½ teaspoon garlic salt
½ cup white vinegar
1 teaspoon dill weed
¼ teaspoon Tabasco sauce
2 tablespoons grated onion
3 1-gram packets Equal (aspartame) sugar substitute

Place all ingredients in a small bowl and beat with a wire whip to blend. Refrigerate until needed but bring back to room temperature before it is used. Shake well before using and serve 2 tablespoons per serving.

Nutritive values per serving:	CAL	CHO (gm)	PRO (gm)	FAT (gm)	NA (mg)
	29	3	negl.	2	167

Food exchanges per serving: 2 tablespoons free (¼ cup equals 1 vegetable, 1 fat)

Low-sodium diets: Omit salt. Use low-sodium tomato sauce and ¼ teaspoon garlic powder instead of garlic salt.

THOUSAND ISLAND DRESSING

Yields 2¼ cups—18 servings

½ cup Kay's Cooked Dressing (see index)
¼ cup chopped, drained canned pimientos
½ cup chopped, drained dill pickles
2 tablespoons chopped fresh green peppers
¼ cup chili sauce
¼ cup catsup
4 1-gram packets Equal (aspartame) sugar substitute

Place all ingredients in a bowl and mix with a fork until smooth. Place in a covered container and refrigerate until served using 2 tablespoons per serving.

Nutritive values per serving:	CAL	CHO (gm)	PRO (gm)	FAT (gm)	NA (mg)
	21	3	1	1	190

Food exchanges per serving: ½ vegetable
Low-sodium diets: Use salt-free catsup and chili sauce. Use low-sodium variation of Kay's Cooked Dressing.

VINAIGRETTE DRESSING

Yields 3 cups—24 servings

This recipe, which Frances Nielsen makes often, is a great favorite with our families. It is good on tossed salads, vegetables, cold meats, and fish. It is best if you make it fresh when you need it, but it can be refrigerated and then brought back to room temperature for serving, if that is more convenient for you.

½ **cup vegetable oil**
1 **cup vinegar**
1 **tablespoon soy sauce**
1 **tablespoon chopped parsley**
1 **tablespoon chopped celery**
⅓ **cup finely chopped onions**
1 **cup water**
Sugar substitute equal to ½ **cup sugar**
½ **teaspoon vanilla**
¼ **teaspoon garlic powder**

Place all ingredients in a 1-quart container and shake well to mix. Shake well before using. Serve 2 tablespoons per serving.

Nutritive values per serving:	CAL	CHO (gm)	PRO (gm)	FAT (gm)	NA (mg)
	43	1	negl.	5	55

Food exchanges per serving: 1 fat
Low-sodium diets: May be used as written.

YOGURT TOPPING

Yields 1¼ cups—10 servings

I didn't really know where to include this recipe in the book. My neighbor Jan Franks gave me the recipe and it is a good dip, a good salad dressing, and makes a tasty topping for baked potatoes. It is easy to make and keeps well in the refrigerator for a week or more.

2 teaspoons dehydrated minced onions
½ teaspoon salt
1 tablespoon dried parsley flakes
⅛ teaspoon garlic powder
1 cup (8 ounces) plain low-fat yogurt
¼ cup Kay's Cooked Dressing (see index)

Stir together onions, salt, parsley, and garlic powder to blend well in a small bowl. Add yogurt and dressing to dry ingredients and mix lightly but thoroughly. Refrigerate until needed. Serve with fresh vegetables as a dip or a dressing, or as a topping for baked potatoes. Serve 2 tablespoons per serving.

Nutritional values per serving:	CAL	CHO (gm)	PRO (gm)	FAT (gm)	NA (mg)
	19	2	1	1	136

Food exchanges per serving: 2 tablespoons may be considered free (¼ cup is 1 vegetable)

Low-sodium diets: Omit salt. Use low-sodium variation of salad dressing.

13
BREADS

I have always enjoyed making bread and I particularly like to do so now that I'm diabetic. I'm not about to waste my precious bread exchanges. I want to get something really good with them—preferably with fiber, if possible. You can, of course, buy some very good high-fiber breads and if you don't like to bake that is the way to go. However, if you like to make breads, I'm sure you will enjoy making bread suitable for your diet.

It isn't terribly difficult to find a good bread when you are diabetic, but if it must also be suitable for a low-cholesterol diet, you need to be more careful in your selection. You want to be sure that the bread you buy doesn't include any whole milk, egg yolks, butter, or most shortenings. French, Italian, and Vienna bread are traditionally suitable because they are generally made of flour, oil, water, and a little salt. However, unless you live in or near a city it can be difficult to find them.

It isn't advisable to buy many of the specialty breads in bakeries if you are on a low-cholesterol diet, because most bakeries won't give you a list of the ingredients in their specialty breads. They may not have sugar in them but they might have egg yolks or some other no-nos. Many of the light commercial breads are safe because they contain dry milk and oil for reasons of cost, but if you do buy them be sure to read the list of ingredients on the wrapper. Remember, the ingredients are listed in the order of their importance, so the first ingredients on the list are always the ones that form the greatest percentage of the final product.

I've never been able to understand why salt-free bread is so expensive and so scarce. It doesn't cost any more to make than regular bread. Maybe it is because they sell less of it and don't want to bother with it. If you need salt-free bread, it is easy to make one of your favorite recipes using oil or salt-free margarine for the fat, and without salt and other ingredients such as milk and cheese which are high in sodium. Most of the breads in this chapter are low in sodium, and those that aren't can easily be adapted for a low-sodium diet. Salt gives flavor to bread but you can always use salt substitute or add some flavoring such as herbs, spices, or seeds like caraway or sesame if you feel the need for more flavor. I like to add a little cinnamon to low-sodium whole grain bread—not enough to make it taste like cinnamon, but just enough to give it a little flavor, about ¼ teaspoon per loaf. You can also add some sugar substitute to give it a slightly sweet taste that helps compensate for not using salt.

Making bread isn't all that difficult, but it is important to pay close attention to correct temperatures and ingredients. I use a thermometer every time I make bread to check the temperature of the liquid in which I dissolve the yeast. Using liquid that is too hot or too cold can spoil a batch of bread very quickly. I have a friend (who shall be nameless) who could never make good bread. She was thoroughly discouraged because her husband loved homemade bread. In fact, I used to send him over a loaf of bread occasionally because he was always doing something nice for us. Eventually we got together, and I told her that there must be some little thing she was doing wrong and to tell me exactly how she made her bread. The first thing she told me was that she used water that was just barely lukewarm, as her mother always had—and that explained her failures. Her mother had used the old-fashioned yeast cake and my friend was using active dry yeast. Once we got that straightened out, my friend started using a thermometer to check the temperature of the water before she added the yeast and began making excellent bread.

Flour is a very important part of making bread, and it is a good idea to use a good quality flour. I keep all-purpose and bread flour at room temperature because I use them up fast. However, I keep an assortment of whole grain flours in the refrigerator or freezer, taking care to bring them back to room temperature before I use them, because I don't always use them all that quickly. I like to use bread flour because of its high gluten content, which helps compensate for the lower gluten content of the whole grain flours. However, it does take more liquid than all-purpose flour, and therefore you need to use a recipe specifically written for the bread flour or do some experimenting with it when you are adapting your own recipes. I use whole grain flours whenever possible because I am convinced that a high-fiber regime is good for anyone on a low-cholesterol or diabetic diet.

Instant dry milk is used in many of the recipes because it is convenient, economical, easy to use, and easy to store. It gives me a good feeling to know that if I decide to do some baking unexpectedly, I won't need to run down to the store for milk. Also, using dry milk means you don't need to scald it before you add it to the bread, and that is a timesaver. It is free of butterfat and therefore good for a low-cholesterol diet. I also use dehydrated buttermilk in many of the recipes in this book for the same reasons. I very seldom reconstitute the milk when using it for breads because it can be added very easily along with other dry ingredients, and you get the same results as if you had added water to it and then added it to the dough or batter.

It is also very convenient to use liquid egg substitute instead of egg yolks for the low-cholesterol diet. It can get a little expensive if you use a lot of it so I try to use egg whites whenever possible, but there are some recipes that really need those whole eggs. It is wonderful to have the liquid egg substitute to use when egg whites just can't replace those cholesterol-rich whole eggs.

Many people think yeast needs sugar to grow, but it will thrive without any sugar in the recipe. If you have a recipe that you feel absolutely has to have a couple of tablespoons of sugar, go ahead and use it, but include the sugar in your nutritive calculations.

If you want to use your own recipes for baking bread, you can use them if you calculate them according to the information in Chapter 2. You will probably find you will have to adjust the number of slices in each loaf, but you shouldn't have any other difficulties unless you are using ingredients that are not suitable on a low-sodium or low-cholesterol diet.

I find that I can make a much better loaf of bread using the dough hook on my electric mixer. If you don't have a dough hook, you can do the first step in the regular mixer and then put it all in a big bowl to add the final flour to the batter by hand—or you can do the whole process by hand. If you are doing it by hand, you should knead the dough for several minutes to develop the gluten, since you aren't developing it with the dough hook in the mixer. Our mothers didn't have dough hooks or even mixers sometimes for making bread and they did a very good job without them, but they kneaded the bread for a long time. One friend of my mother's prided herself that she kneaded her bread for a whole hour. I find the thought very tiring (although she did make wonderful bread). However, I think it is unnecessary to knead it for more than a few minutes if you are doing it by hand.

The number of loaves and the slices per loaf are shown with each recipe. This is very important because it is an essential part of the information used to calculate the food exchanges per serving. The diabetic calculations are accurate only if you follow the recipes exactly and then cut the finished product into the number of servings shown on the recipe.

Any loaf of bread can be used to make rolls, if you roll the dough out into a long roll and then cut it into the same number of pieces that you would cut for a finished loaf. Then each portion can be used to make a roll with the same nutritive values as each slice of bread would have contained. If you want larger rolls, cut the bread dough into half the number of pieces you would cut for a finished loaf, and then shape and bake, with each roll having twice the nutritive values of a slice of bread.

Homemade bread has always been a special treat. Since we have lost so many of our special treats because we are diabetic, I believe in providing myself and other diabetics with fresh homemade bread whenever possible. I hope you feel the same way and that you will enjoy preparing these breads for yourself and others.

APPLESAUCE NUT BREAD

Yields 1 loaf—16 servings

⅓ cup (⅔ stick) margarine at room temperature
3 tablespoons sugar
3 large egg whites at room temperature
1 cup all-purpose flour
⅔ cup graham flour
1 teaspoon pumpkin pie spice
1 tablespoon baking powder
½ teaspoon baking soda
½ teaspoon salt
1 cup unsweetened applesauce
Liquid sugar substitute equal to 3 tablespoons sugar
½ cup chopped nuts

Cream margarine and sugar together until light and fluffy. Add egg whites to creamed mixture and beat at medium speed for ½ minute.

Stir together flours, spice, baking powder, soda, and salt until well blended.

Add applesauce, sweetener, and nuts, along with flour mixture, to creamed mixture. Mix at medium speed only until the flour is moistened. Do not overbeat. Spread evenly in a 9" × 5" × 3" loaf pan that has been greased with margarine. Bake at 375° F. for 45 minutes, or until a cake tester comes out clean from the center and the bread pulls away from the sides of the pan. Cool 10 minutes in the pan and turn out onto a wire rack to cool to room temperature. Cut into 16 equal slices. Serve 1 slice per serving.

	CAL	CHO (gm)	PRO (gm)	FAT (gm)	NA (mg)
Nutritive values per serving:	126	15	3	6	183

Food exchanges per serving: 1 bread, 1 fat
Low-sodium diets: Omit salt. Use salt-free margarine and low-sodium baking powder.

BANANA NUT BREAD

Yields 1 loaf—14 servings

This recipe is based on one from Florence Jennings who lives here in Wadena. I've always thought that it was the best banana bread I've ever eaten. It isn't terribly rich but it has a wonderful flavor. Florence is a very good cook—and we also share an interest in quilts and quilting.

½ cup (1 stick) margarine at room temperature
2 tablespoons sugar
½ cup liquid egg substitute at room temperature
Liquid sugar substitute equal to ⅓ cup sugar
1 cup all-purpose flour
¾ cup oat bran
2 teaspoons baking powder
½ teaspoon baking soda
1 cup mashed bananas (3 medium bananas)
¼ cup chopped nuts

Cream together margarine and sugar at medium speed until light and fluffy. Add egg substitute and sweetener to creamed mixture and beat at medium speed for 1 minute.

Stir together flour, oat bran, baking powder, and soda to blend well. Add bananas to creamed mixture along with the flour mixture and beat 1 minute at medium speed.

Add nuts to batter and mix lightly. Spread evenly in a 9" × 5" × 3" loaf pan which has been greased with margarine. Bake at 375° F. for 45 minutes, or until a cake tester comes out clean from the center of the loaf and the loaf starts to pull away from the sides of the pan. Cool in the pan for 10 minutes. Turn out onto a wire rack and cool to room temperature. Cut into 14 equal slices and serve at room temperature. Serve 1 slice per serving.

Nutritive values per serving:	CAL	CHO (gm)	PRO (gm)	FAT (gm)	NA (mg)
	142	16	3	8	173

Food exchanges per serving: 1 bread, 1½ fat
Low-sodium diets: Use salt-free margarine and low-sodium baking powder.

CHOCOLATE NUT BREAD

Yields 1 loaf—16 servings

If you are a chocoholic (and it seems to me that most diabetics are), this bread is for you. Even nondiabetics love it. I like to serve it with peanut butter. It sounds unusual, but chocolate and peanut butter go well together.

1¾ **cups all-purpose flour**
⅓ **cup cocoa**
¼ **cup dry buttermilk**
¼ **cup sugar**
1 **teaspoon cinnamon**
1 **teaspoon baking soda**
1 **teaspoon baking powder**
1 **cup water**
¼ **cup vegetable oil**
¼ **cup liquid egg substitute at room temperature**
Liquid sugar substitute equal to ⅓ **cup sugar**
1 **teaspoon vanilla**
½ **cup chopped nuts**

Place first 7 ingredients in mixer bowl and mix at low speed to blend well.

Mix water, oil, egg substitute, sweetener, and vanilla with a fork to blend. Add to flour mixture and mix at medium speed only until flour is moistened. Do not overbeat.

Add nuts to dough and spread evenly in a 9″ × 5″ × 3″ loaf pan that has been greased with margarine. Bake at 375° F. for 45 minutes or until a cake tester comes out clean from the center and the bread pulls away from the sides of the pan. Let cool in the pan for 10 minutes and then turn out onto a wire rack to cool to room temperature. Cut into 16 equal slices. Serve 1 slice per serving.

Nutritive values per serving:	CAL	CHO (gm)	PRO (gm)	FAT (gm)	NA (mg)
	131	16	4	6	104

Food exchanges per serving: 1 bread, 1 fat
Low-sodium diets: Use low-sodium baking powder.

ZUCCHINI BREAD

Yields 1 loaf—18 servings

This recipe is based on one from Delores LeMaster of Strawberry Point, Iowa. Delores, who is also diabetic, works at the nursing home where I work as a dietary consultant. She is quite clever about adapting recipes for her own use and she often shares them with me.

2 cups all-purpose flour
1½ teaspoons cinnamon
¼ teaspoon salt
1 teaspoon baking soda
½ teaspoon baking powder
3 large egg whites
⅓ cup vegetable oil
1½ teaspoons vanilla
1½ tablespoons Sweet-10
1½ cups well-packed shredded fresh zucchini

Place flour, cinnamon, salt, soda, and baking powder in a mixer bowl and mix at low speed to blend well.

Place egg whites, oil, vanilla, and sweetener in a cup and mix well with a fork to blend.

Add zucchini to flour mixture along with oil mixture and mix at medium speed until well blended and creamy. Pour into a 9″ × 5″ × 3″ loaf pan that has been greased with margarine. Bake at 375° F. for 45 minutes, or until a cake tester comes out clean from the center and the bread pulls away from the sides of the pan. Cool in the pan for 10 minutes. Turn out onto a wire rack and cool to room temperature. Cut into 18 equal slices and serve 1 slice per serving.

Nutritive values per serving:	CAL	CHO (gm)	PRO (gm)	FAT (gm)	NA (mg)
	91	11	2	4	104

Food exchanges per serving: 1 fruit, 1 fat
Low-sodium diets: Omit salt. Use low-sodium baking powder.

BRAN NUT MUFFINS

Yields 12 muffins—12 servings

1 cup water
1 cup All Bran, Bran Buds, 100% Bran, or oat bran
Liquid sugar substitute equal to 3 tablespoons sugar (optional)
2 large egg whites at room temperature
⅓ cup (⅔ stick) margarine at room temperature
1¼ cups all-purpose flour
¼ cup instant dry milk
4 teaspoons baking powder
¼ cup chopped nuts

Combine water, bran, sweetener, and egg whites and let sit for 5 to 10 minutes.

Cream margarine at medium speed until light and fluffy.

Stir flour, dry milk, baking powder, and nuts to blend well and add to creamed margarine along with bran mixture. Mix at medium speed only until flour is moistened. Do not overmix. Grease muffin tins with margarine or line with paper liners. Fill muffin tins half full and bake at 400° F. for 20 to 25 minutes or until muffins spring back when touched in the center. Serve hot, if possible. Serve 1 muffin per serving.

Nutritive values per serving:	CAL	CHO (gm)	PRO (gm)	FAT (gm)	NA (mg)
	133	15	4	7	274

Food exchanges per serving: 1 bread, 1 fat
Low-sodium diets: Use salt-free margarine and low-sodium baking powder.

DARK BRAN MUFFINS

Yields 12 muffins—12 servings

1 cup all-purpose flour
1 teaspoon baking soda
1 cup All Bran, Bran Buds, 100% Bran, or oat bran
¼ cup dry buttermilk
1 cup water
2 large egg whites at room temperature
2 tablespoons vegetable oil
Liquid sugar substitute equal to 3 tablespoons sugar (optional)
¼ cup dark molasses

Place flour, soda, bran, and dry buttermilk in mixer bowl and mix at low speed to blend.

Combine water, egg whites, oil, sweetener, and molasses and stir with a fork to blend. Add to flour mixture and mix at medium speed only until flour is moistened. Grease muffin tins with margarine or line with paper liners. Fill muffin tins half full and bake at 400° F. for 20 to 25 minutes, or until muffins spring back when touched in the center. Serve hot, if possible. Serve 1 muffin per serving.

Nutritive values per serving:

CAL	CHO (gm)	PRO (gm)	FAT (gm)	NA (mg)
97	17	3	3	154

Food exchanges per serving: 1 bread, ½ fat
Low-sodium diets: The recipe may be used as written.

RAISIN BRAN MUFFINS

Yields 12 muffins—12 servings

1 cup water
2 large egg whites at room temperature
¼ cup vegetable oil
¼ cup instant dry milk
1 cup all-purpose flour
1 tablespoon baking powder
1 cup All Bran, Bran Buds, 100% Bran, or oat bran
¼ cup raisins

Place water, egg whites, oil, and dry milk in mixer bowl and mix at low speed to blend.

Stir together flour and baking powder to blend.

Add bran and raisins to liquid along with flour mixture. Mix at medium speed only until flour is moistened. Do not overmix. Grease muffin tins with margarine or line with paper liners. Fill muffin tins half full and bake at 400° F. for 20 to 25 minutes, or until muffins spring back when touched in the center. Serve hot, if possible. Serve 1 muffin per serving.

Nutritive values per serving:	CAL	CHO (gm)	PRO (gm)	FAT (gm)	NA (mg)
	107	15	3	5	166

Food exchanges per serving: 1 bread, 1 fat
Low-sodium diets: Use low-sodium baking powder.

REFRIGERATOR BRAN MUFFINS

Yields 30 muffins—30 servings

This recipe is based on one from Doris Walker of Grinnell, Iowa. Doris and her husband Denver lived in Wadena when we first moved here, but returned back home to Grinnell when they retired. I like to keep this batter on hand and generally bake 6 of them at a time. They are a dark, rich muffin which I often serve to friends without telling them they are a low-sugar recipe.

3 cups Bran Buds, All Bran, or 100% Bran
3 cups water
⅓ cup vegetable oil
4 large egg whites
Liquid sugar substitute equal to ⅓ cup sugar
2½ cups all-purpose flour
½ cup dry buttermilk
¼ cup sugar
1 tablespoon soda
½ teaspoon salt

Place bran, water, oil, egg whites, and sweetener in mixer bowl and mix at low speed to blend.

Stir remaining dry ingredients together to blend well. Add to bran mixture and mix at medium speed only to blend. Line 30 muffin tins with paper cups or spray with pan spray. Fill muffin tins about ½ full and bake at 375° F. for about 20 minutes, or until they spring back when touched in the center. Serve hot if possible, 1 muffin per serving.

Muffins can be baked immediately or batter can be covered and kept in the refrigerator for up to 3 weeks. The batter does not need to be brought to room temperature when it is used. If the batter gets too thick, it can be thinned with a little hot water.

Nutritive values per serving:	CAL	CHO (gm)	PRO (gm)	FAT (gm)	NA (mg)
	90	15	3	3	205

Food exchanges per serving: 1 bread, ½ fat
Low-sodium diets: Omit salt.

APPLESAUCE OAT BRAN MUFFINS

Yields 12 muffins—12 servings

1 cup all-purpose flour
1 cup oat bran
¼ cup packed brown sugar
4 teaspoons baking powder
1 teaspoon ground cinnamon or pumpkin pie spice
½ cup unsweetened applesauce
½ cup water
¼ cup vegetable oil
2 large egg whites

Place flour, oat bran, brown sugar, baking powder, and cinnamon or pumpkin pie spice in bowl and mix well at low speed. In a separate bowl combine applesauce, water, oil, and egg whites and beat with a fork to blend.

Add applesauce mixture to flour mixture and mix at medium speed only until all flour is moistened. Grease muffin tins with margarine or line with paper cups. Fill muffin tins ½ full and bake at 400° F. for about 20 minutes, or until muffins are browned and spring back when touched in the center. Serve hot, if possible, using 1 muffin per serving.

Nutritive values per serving:	CAL	CHO (gm)	PRO (gm)	FAT (gm)	NA (mg)
	120	18	3	5	120
Food exchanges per serving:	1 bread, 1 fat				
Low-sodium diets:	This recipe may be used as written.				

CHOCOLATE OAT BRAN MUFFINS

Yields 12 muffins—12 servings

These muffins can add more variety to the oat bran muffins you take along to work for coffee breaks. If you want them sweeter, you can add two teaspoons dry Weight Watchers sugar substitute along with the flour without changing the food exchange value.

1 cup all-purpose flour
1 cup oat bran
⅓ cup cocoa
¼ cup sugar
1 tablespoon baking powder
½ teaspoon salt
1 cup plus 2 tablespoons water at room temperature
¼ cup vegetable oil
2 large egg whites
1 teaspoon vanilla

Place flour, oat bran, cocoa, sugar, baking powder, and salt in a mixer bowl and mix well at low speed. Combine water, oil, egg whites, and vanilla and stir with a fork to blend.

Add liquid mixture to flour mixture and mix at low speed only until all flour is moistened. Grease muffin tins with margarine or line with paper cups. Fill muffin tins ½ full and bake at 400° F. for about 20 minutes, or until muffins spring back when touched in the center. Serve hot, if possible, using 1 muffin per serving.

Nutritive values per serving:

CAL	CHO (gm)	PRO (gm)	FAT (gm)	NA (mg)
106	15	4	5	176

Food exchanges per serving: 1 bread, 1 fat
Low-sodium diets: Omit salt. Use low-sodium baking powder.

CINNAMON APPLESAUCE MUFFINS

Yields 12 muffins—12 servings

I like to have a variety of oat and wheat bran muffins in the freezer so that I can have a different kind to pop in the microwave for breakfast each morning or with a salad or soup for lunch.

1 cup 100% Bran
2 large egg whites
¼ cup vegetable oil
1 cup unsweetened applesauce
2 tablespoons brown sugar
2 tablespoons water
1 cup all-purpose flour
1 teaspoon Weight Watchers dry sugar substitute (optional)
1 teaspoon soda
2 tablespoons dry buttermilk
½ teaspoon salt
1 teaspoon ground cinnamon

Place bran, egg whites, oil, applesauce, brown sugar, and water in mixer bowl. Mix lightly to blend and let sit at room temperature for 30–45 minutes.
Stir flour, sugar substitute, soda, dry buttermilk, salt, and cinnamon together to blend well. Add to bran mixture and mix at medium speed only until all flour is moistened. Grease muffin tins with margarine or line with paper cups. Fill tins about ½ full and bake at 400° F. for 20 minutes, or until muffins spring back when touched in the center. Serve hot if possible.

Nutritive values per serving:	CAL	CHO (gm)	PRO (gm)	FAT (gm)	NA (mg)
	116	17	5	3	181

Food exchanges per serving: 1 bread, 1 fat
Low-sodium diets: Omit salt.

YANKEE CORNBREAD

Yields 1 9-inch square—16 servings

If you like your cornbread thicker, bake it in an 8-inch square pan. I like it thinner and crustier so we bake it in a 9-inch square pan—and we bake it often because my husband thinks that cornbread goes along with almost anything.

1 cup cornmeal
1 cup all-purpose flour
4 teaspoons baking powder
¼ cup sugar
¼ cup instant dry milk
¼ teaspoon salt
1 cup water at room temperature
¼ cup liquid egg substitute at room temperature
¼ cup vegetable oil

Place dry ingredients in mixer bowl and mix at low speed to blend well. (I find that I get much better results mixing it in a mixer than I do when I mix it by hand.)

Beat together water, egg substitute, and oil with a fork and add all at once to the flour mixture. Beat at low speed only until the flour is moistened. Pour into an 8- or 9-inch pan that has been greased with margarine. Bake at 400° F. for about 25 minutes for a 9-inch pan or 30–35 minutes for an 8-inch pan. Serve hot, if possible. Cut 4 × 4 to yield 16 squares. Serve 1 square per serving.

Nutritive values per serving:

	CAL	CHO (gm)	PRO (gm)	FAT (gm)	NA (mg)
	110	17	2	4	126

Food exchanges per serving: 1 bread, 1 fat
Low-sodium diets: Omit salt. Use low-sodium baking powder.

GRAHAM SCONES

Yields 1 9-inch round—16 servings

Scones can be, and often are, made from all-white flour, but I like to think that this is more like the way they were made in Scotland before white flour was so readily available.

1 cup graham flour
1 cup all-purpose flour
4 teaspoons baking powder
2 tablespoons brown sugar
1 teaspoon cinnamon
¼ teaspoon salt
½ cup (1 stick) margarine
¼ cup raisins or currants
¼ cup liquid egg substitute at room temperature
⅔ cup skim milk

Place flours, baking powder, sugar, cinnamon, and salt in a mixing bowl and stir with a spoon to blend well. Cut margarine into the flour mixture with a pastry blender until it resembles coarse meal. Stir raisins or currants into the flour and margarine mixture to coat them with flour.

Mix together egg substitute and milk and add as much as necessary of the mixture to the flour mixture to make a soft dough like a baking powder biscuit dough. Knead several times in the bowl and then turn out onto a lightly floured working surface. Shape into a 9-inch round and place on a baking sheet which has been lightly greased with margarine. Crease the top of the round about ¼ inch deep to form 16 equal pie-shaped wedges. The scones may be baked as they are or the wedges may be cut through and separated to form a crustier scone. If left whole, the scones should be baked at 400° F. for 25–30 minutes, then broken apart and served hot. If separated, the wedges should be baked at 400° F. about 15 minutes or until browned and crisp. Serve 1 wedge per serving

Nutritive values per serving:	CAL	CHO (gm)	PRO (gm)	FAT (gm)	NA (mg)
	124	16	3	6	198

Food exchanges per serving: 1 bread, 1 fat
Low-sodium diets: Omit salt. Use low-sodium baking powder and salt-free margarine.

CHALLAH

Yields 2 loaves—40 servings

This Jewish bread makes marvelous French toast or bread pudding if you have any of it left over.

1⅓ **cups water at 110–115° F.**
2 packages (1½ tablespoons) active dry yeast
7 cups all-purpose flour, divided
1 cup liquid egg substitute at room temperature
2 teaspoons salt
¼ **cup (½ stick) margarine at room temperature**
1 egg white at room temperature
¼ **cup water at room temperature**
2 teaspoons sesame seeds

Place water and yeast in mixer bowl. Mix lightly and let set for 5 minutes. Add 3 cups flour to liquid and beat at low speed, using dough hook, for 4 minutes.

Add egg substitute, salt, margarine, and 3 cups flour to dough and mix, using dough hook, at low speed for another 2 minutes or until a smooth dough is formed.

Turn dough out onto a working surface and knead, using as much of the remaining flour as necessary to form a smooth resilient dough. Form into a ball and place in a bowl that has been well greased with margarine. Turn the ball over to cover the top with margarine. Cover and let stand in a warm place until doubled in volume.

Turn dough out onto a lightly floured working surface and knead lightly. Form into a ball and return to the bowl, turning the ball over to grease the top of it. Cover and let rise until doubled in volume.

Turn the dough out onto a lightly floured working surface. Divide the dough into 2 equal portions. Round each portion into a ball. Cover with a cloth and let rest for 10 minutes. Divide each ball into 3 equal portions. Roll each portion gently to form a roll about 14 inches long. Braid 3 rolls to form a loaf. Place the loaves on 1 or 2 cookie sheets that have been greased lightly with margarine. Cover with a cloth and let stand in a warm place until doubled in volume.

Beat egg white and water together with a fork until smooth. Brush each loaf with the egg white mixture and sprinkle with sesame seeds. Bake at 400° F. for 30 minutes or until the loaves sound hollow and are lightly browned. Transfer loaves to wire rack to cool to room temperature. Cut each loaf into 20 equal slices and serve 1 slice per serving.

Nutritive values per serving:	CAL	CHO (gm)	PRO (gm)	FAT (gm)	NA (mg)
	97	17	3	2	132

Food exchanges per serving: 1 bread
Low-sodium diets: Omit salt. Use salt-free margarine.

Note: This bread can be baked in regular loaf pans, if desired. If the dough is baked in 3 equal loaves and each loaf is cut into 14 slices, each slice will provide the following:

Nutritive values per serving:	CAL	CHO (gm)	PRO (gm)	FAT (gm)	NA (mg)
	92	16	3	2	125

Food exchanges per serving: 1 bread

WHOLE WHEAT ITALIAN BREAD

Yields 2 loaves—36 servings

This bread dough makes excellent hard rolls. We like to divide the dough into 18 equal portions, shape it into long hard rolls, and bake them to eat with hot beef sandwiches. Each roll is equal to 2 bread exchanges with double the nutritive values for each slice of bread.

2 cups water at 110–115° F.
2 packages (1½ tablespoons) active dry yeast
4 cups all-purpose flour
¼ cup vegetable oil
2 teaspoons salt
2 cups whole wheat flour, divided
1 egg white
1 tablespoon cold water

Combine water and yeast and let stand 5 minutes in mixer bowl. Add 4 cups all-purpose flour to liquid and beat 4 minutes at medium speed, using dough hook. Add oil, salt, and 1½ cups whole wheat flour to batter and beat, using dough hook, at low speed for 4 minutes.

Use as much of the remaining flour as necessary to make a smooth, resilient loaf. Turn dough out onto a lightly floured working surface and knead a few times. Form into a ball and place in a bowl that has been greased with margarine. Cover with a cloth and set in a warm place until doubled in volume.

Turn dough out onto a lightly floured working surface. Knead about 2 minutes. Form into a ball and return to greased bowl. Turn the ball over to coat the top of it with margarine. Cover and set in a warm place until doubled in volume.

Turn dough out onto a lightly floured working surface, knead lightly, and divide into 2 equal portions. Form each portion into a ball and let rest, covered with a cloth, for 10 minutes. Shape each roll into a long, thin loaf tapered at the end. Place loaves diagonally, seamed side down, on greased baking sheets. Cut slits about ⅛-inch deep, about 2 inches apart on tops of loaves.

Beat egg white and 1 tablespoon water together and brush tops and sides of loaves with this mixture. Cover with a cloth and let rise again until doubled in volume.

Bake at 400° F. for 10 minutes; reduce heat to 350° F. and bake another 10 minutes. Brush tops and sides of loaves again with egg white mixture. Continue baking for another 30 minutes for a total of 50 minutes, or until loaves are golden brown. Turn out on a wire rack and cool to room temperature. Cut each loaf into 18 equal slices and serve 1 slice per serving.

Nutritive values per serving:	CAL	CHO (gm)	PRO (gm)	FAT (gm)	NA (mg)
	88	15	3	2	119

Food exchanges per serving: 1 bread
Low-sodium diets: Omit salt.

RAISIN BREAD

Yields 2 loaves—36 servings

I have always loved raisin bread. I just wish that raisins weren't so high in carbohydrate so we could double the amount of them in the bread.

1½ cups hot water .
⅓ cup instant dry milk
2 packages (1½ tablespoons) active dry yeast
5 cups all-purpose flour, divided
Liquid sugar substitute equal to ½ cup sugar (optional)
2 teaspoons salt
¼ cup liquid egg substitute at room temperature
¼ cup vegetable oil
½ cup raisins

Place water and dry milk in mixer bowl and mix at slow speed only to dissolve milk. Let cool to 110–115° F. Add yeast to liquid and let stand for 5 minutes. Add 2 cups flour to liquid and mix at low speed, using dough hook, for 3 minutes.

Add sweetener, salt, egg substitute, oil, and 2 cups flour to batter and mix at low speed, using dough hook, for another 2 minutes. Add raisins to dough and mix at low speed for another minute.

Turn dough out onto a working surface spread with 1 cup flour and knead, using as much of the remaining flour as necessary to form a smooth, elastic dough. Form dough into a ball and place in a bowl which has been well greased with margarine. Turn the ball over so the top will be greased with the margarine, cover, and let stand in a warm place until doubled in volume.

Turn dough out onto a lightly floured working surface and knead lightly. Form into a ball and return to the greased bowl, turning the top of the ball over so it will be greased on top. Cover and let stand in a warm place until doubled in volume.

Turn the dough out onto a lightly floured working surface. Knead lightly. Divide into 2 equal parts. Form each half into a ball, cover, and let rest for 10 minutes. Form each ball into a loaf and place each loaf in a 9″ × 5″ × 3″ loaf pan that has been greased with margarine. Cover and let rise in a warm place until doubled in volume.

Bake at 375° F. for about 45 minutes or until browned. As soon as the bread is removed from the oven, turn it out onto a wire rack and brush it with margarine. Slice each loaf into 18 equal slices and serve 1 slice per serving.

Nutritive values per serving:	CAL	CHO (gm)	PRO (gm)	FAT (gm)	NA (mg)
	89	15	3	2	125

Food exchanges per serving: 1 bread
Low-sodium diets: Omit salt.

COUNTRY LOAF

Yields 3 loaves—42 servings

This bread is also good for a low-sodium diet. Without the salt, it contains only 3 mg sodium per serving.

2½ cups hot water
2 tablespoons brown sugar
1 cup cornmeal
2 packages (1½ tablespoons) active dry yeast
3½ cups bread flour, divided
¼ cup liquid egg substitute
¼ cup vegetable oil
2 teaspoons salt
2 cups graham or whole wheat flour

Place water, sugar, and cornmeal in a mixer bowl. Mix to dissolve the sugar and let cool to 110–115° F. Add yeast to liquid mixture and let stand for 5 minutes. Add 3 cups bread flour to liquid and beat at medium speed, using dough hook, for 4 minutes. Add egg substitute, oil, salt, and 2 cups graham flour to batter and beat at low speed, using dough hook, for another 4 minutes.

Use as much of the remaining bread flour as necessary to make a smooth, resilient loaf. Turn dough out onto a lightly floured working surface and knead a couple of times. Form into a ball and place in a bowl that has been greased with margarine. Turn the ball over to coat the top of it with margarine. Cover with a cloth and set in a warm place until doubled in volume.

Turn dough out onto a lightly floured working surface and knead lightly. Form into a ball and return to greased bowl. Turn the ball over to coat the top with margarine. Cover with a cloth and set in a warm place until doubled in volume.

Turn dough out onto a lightly floured working surface, knead lightly, and divide into 3 equal portions. Form each portion into a ball and let rest, covered with a cloth, for 10 minutes. Form each ball into a loaf and place in a 9" × 5" × 3" loaf pan that has been greased with margarine.

Cover and let rise until doubled in volume. Bake at 475° F. for 45 minutes or until browned and firm. Turn out onto a wire rack and cool to room temperature. Cut each loaf into 14 equal slices and serve 1 slice per serving.

Nutritive values per serving:	CAL	CHO (gm)	PRO (gm)	FAT (gm)	NA (mg)
	88	16	2	2	105
Food exchanges per serving:	1 bread				
Low-sodium diets:	Omit salt.				

RICH WHOLE WHEAT BREAD

Yields 3 loaves—42 servings

This is a good bread for a low-sodium diet. Without the salt, it contains only 3 mg sodium per slice. However, I included the salt because if you aren't on a low-sodium diet, it adds to the flavor of the bread.

2 cups hot water
¼ cup brown sugar
2 packages (1½ tablespoons) active dry yeast
3½ cups bread flour, divided
⅓ cup vegetable oil
¼ cup liquid egg substitute
2 teaspoons salt
3 cups whole wheat flour

Place water and sugar in mixer bowl and stir to dissolve sugar. Cool to 110–115° F. Add yeast to liquid and let stand for 5 minutes. Add 3 cups bread flour to liquid and mix, using dough hook, for 4 minutes at medium speed.

Add oil, egg substitute, salt, and 3 cups whole wheat flour to dough and mix, using dough hook, for 4 minutes at low speed.

Add as much of the remaining bread flour as necessary to the dough to make a smooth, resilient dough. Turn out onto a lightly floured working surface and knead a few times. Form into a ball and place in a bowl that has been greased with margarine. Turn the ball over to coat the top of the ball with margarine. Cover with a cloth and set in a warm place until doubled in volume.

Turn dough out onto a lightly floured working surface and knead lightly. Form into a ball and return to the greased bowl. Turn the ball over to coat the top of it with margarine. Cover with a cloth and set in a warm place until doubled in volume.

Turn dough out onto a lightly floured working surface, knead lightly, and divide into 3 equal portions. Form each portion into a ball and let rest, covered with a cloth, for 10 minutes. Form each ball into a loaf and place each loaf in a 9" × 5" × 3" loaf pan that has been greased with margarine. Cover and let rise in a warm place until doubled in volume. Bake at 375° F. for 45 minutes, or until browned and firm. Turn bread out onto wire rack and let cool to room temperature. Cut each loaf into 14 equal slices and serve 1 slice per serving.

Nutritive values per serving:	CAL	CHO (gm)	PRO (gm)	FAT (gm)	NA (mg)
	97	17	3	2	105

Food exchanges per serving: 1 bread
Low-sodium diets: Omit salt.

PANETTONE

Yields 1 loaf—18 servings

This bread has been a favorite of mine since Chuck's cousin sent us a loaf from Milan, Italy, as a Christmas gift one year. I tried to duplicate it but couldn't until I added anise flavoring and used bread flour. It is frequently baked in a round shape on a cookie sheet or in a special panettone pan that I have, but it is easier to cut into the right portions when it is baked in a loaf pan.

¾ **cup water at 110–115° F.**
2 tablespoons instant dry milk
1 package (2¼ teaspoons) active dry yeast
2¼ cups bread flour, divided
Liquid sugar substitute equal to 3 tablespoons sugar
2 drops yellow food coloring
¼ **teaspoon anise extract**
⅛ **teaspoon ground ginger**
¼ **cup liquid egg substitute at room temperature**
½ **teaspoon salt**
2 tablespoons margarine at room temperature
¼ **cup chopped candied cherries**

Combine water, dry milk, and yeast and let stand for 5 minutes in a mixer bowl. Add 1 cup flour to liquid and beat at low speed, using a dough hook, for 4 minutes.

Add sweetener, food coloring, anise, ginger, egg substitute, salt, margarine, and 1 cup flour to batter and mix at low speed, using a dough hook, for another 4 minutes. Add candied cherries to dough and mix, using a dough hook, only until fruit is mixed into the dough.

Use as much additional flour as necessary to form a smooth, resilient loaf. Turn dough out onto lightly floured working surface and knead a couple of times. Form into a ball and place in a bowl that has been well greased with margarine. Turn the ball over to coat the top of it with margarine. Cover with a cloth and set in a warm place until doubled in volume.

Turn dough out onto a lightly floured working surface and knead lightly. Form into a ball and return to greased bowl, turning the top again to coat it with margarine. Cover with a cloth and set in a warm place until doubled in volume.

Turn dough out onto a lightly floured working surface, knead lightly, and form into a ball. Cover with a cloth and let rest for 10 minutes. Form into a loaf and place in a 9" × 5" × 3" loaf pan that has been greased with margarine. Cover and let rise again until doubled in volume. Bake at 375° F for 45 minutes until well browned and firm. Turn out onto a wire rack and cool to room temperature. Cut into 18 equal slices and serve 1 slice per serving.

Note: It is important to use bread flour in this recipe. However, if you do use all-purpose flour (3¼ cups) and cut each loaf into 18 equal slices, each slice will have a nutritive value of 1⅓ bread exchanges (114 calories); or you can cut it into 24 thin slices with a nutritive value of 1 bread exchange (85 calories) per serving.

Nutritive values per serving:	CAL	CHO (gm)	PRO (gm)	FAT (gm)	NA (mg)
	97	18	3	2	82

Food exchanges per serving of basic recipe: 1 bread

Low-sodium diets: Omit salt. Use salt-free margarine.

THREE-GRAIN BREAD

Yields 2 loaves—36 servings

½ **cup cornmeal**
2 teaspoons salt
¼ **cup (½ stick) margarine**
2 cups boiling water
2 packages (1½ tablespoons) active dry yeast
½ **cup water at 110–115° F.**
3 cups bread flour, divided
1 cup light rye flour
1 cup graham flour

Place cornmeal, salt, margarine, and 2 cups boiling water in mixer bowl and mix at low speed to melt margarine. Cool to room temperature. Stir together yeast and ½ cup warm water and let rest for 5 minutes. Add to lukewarm mixture and mix lightly. Add 2¾ cups bread flour to liquid mixture and mix at medium speed, using dough hook, for 4 minutes. Add rye and graham flours to dough and mix, using dough hook, for another 4 minutes at low speed.

Spread on working surface. Turn dough out onto working surface and knead, using as much of the remaining bread flour as necessary to form a smooth, resilient dough. Form into a ball and place in a bowl that has been greased with margarine, turning the dough so it is greased on top. Cover with a cloth and let rise in a warm place until it is doubled in volume.

Turn dough out onto a lightly floured working surface and knead lightly. Form into a ball and return to the bowl, turning the ball over to grease the top of it. Cover and let rise until doubled in volume.

Turn the dough out onto a lightly floured working surface. Divide the dough into 2 equal portions. Round each portion into a ball. Cover with a cloth and let rest for 10 minutes. Shape each ball into a loaf and place each loaf in a 9" × 5" × 3" loaf pan that has been greased with margarine. Cover and let rise until doubled in volume. Bake at 375° F. for 45 minutes, or until browned and firm. Turn bread out onto wire rack and let cool to room temperature. Cut each loaf into 18 equal slices and serve 1 slice per serving.

Note: It is important to use bread flour in this recipe. However, if you use all-purpose flour (3¾ cups) and cut each loaf into 18 equal slices, each slice will have a nutritive value of 1 bread exchange (88 calories).

	CAL	CHO (gm)	PRO (gm)	FAT (gm)	NA (mg)
Nutritive values per serving:	82	15	2	2	135

Food exchanges per serving of basic recipe: 1 bread

Low-sodium diets: Omit salt. Use salt-free margarine.

WHOLE WHEAT BREAD

Yields 2 loaves—36 servings

2½ cups water at 110–115° F.
½ cup instant dry milk
2 packages (1½ tablespoons) active dry yeast
3 cups bread flour
¼ cup (½ stick) margarine at room temperature
2 teaspoons salt
2¾ cups whole wheat flour, divided

Combine water, dry milk, and yeast and let stand 5 minutes in a mixer bowl. Add 3 cups bread flour to liquid and beat at medium speed, using dough hook, for 4 minutes.

Add margarine, salt, and 2½ cups whole wheat flour to batter and mix at low speed, using dough hook, for another 4 minutes.

Use as much of the remaining whole wheat flour as necessary to make a smooth, resilient loaf. Turn dough out onto a lightly floured working surface and knead a couple of times. Form into a ball and place in a bowl that has been well greased with margarine. Turn the ball over to coat the top of it with margarine. Cover with a cloth and set in a warm place until doubled in volume.

Turn dough out onto a lightly floured working surface and knead lightly. Form into a ball and return to greased bowl. Turn the ball over to coat the top of it with margarine. Cover with a cloth and set in a warm place until doubled in volume.

Turn dough out onto a lightly floured working surface, knead lightly, and divide into 2 equal portions. Form each portion into a ball and let rest, covered with a cloth, for 10 minutes. Form each ball into a loaf and place in a 9" × 5" × 3" loaf pan that has been greased with margarine. Cover and let rise again until doubled in volume. Bake at 375° F. for 45 minutes, or until browned and firm. Turn out onto a wire rack and cool to room temperature. Cut each loaf into 18 equal slices and serve 1 slice per serving.

Note: It is important to use bread flour in this recipe. The gluten in the bread flour helps give texture to the finished loaf of bread.

Nutritive values per serving:	CAL	CHO (gm)	PRO (gm)	FAT (gm)	NA (mg)
	89	15	2	2	139

Food exchanges per serving: 1 bread
Low-sodium diets: Omit salt. Use salt-free margarine.

CINNAMON ROLLS

Yields 24 rolls—24 servings

These rolls are a great favorite of John Franks, who lives next door to us. I've known him to eat four of them at one time, washed down with a couple of glasses of milk. John is only eight but he knows what he likes for between-meal snacks, and I agree with him that there is nothing like a hot, fresh cinnamon roll, right from the oven.

1 cup water at 110–115° F.
¼ cup instant dry milk
1 package (2¼ teaspoons) active dry yeast
3½ cups all-purpose flour, divided
⅛ teaspoon ground ginger
¼ cup vegetable oil
1 teaspoon salt
1 teaspoon cinnamon (optional)
Liquid sugar substitute equal to 2 tablespoons sugar (optional)
1½ teaspoons margarine at room temperature
½ cup Brown Sugar Twin granulated sugar substitute
1½ tablespoons margarine at room temperature

Place water, dry milk, and yeast in mixer bowl; mix lightly and let set for 5 minutes. Add 1½ cups flour to liquid. Mix at medium speed, using dough hook, for 4 minutes. Add ginger, oil, salt, cinnamon, sweetener, and 1½ cups flour to batter and mix at low speed, using dough hook, for another 4 minutes.

Use as much of the remaining flour as necessary to make a smooth, resilient dough. Shape the dough into a ball and place in a bowl that has been well greased with margarine. Turn the ball over to coat the top with margarine. Cover with a cloth and set in a warm place until doubled in volume.

Turn dough out onto a lightly floured working surface and knead lightly. Form into a ball and return to greased bowl, turning the top again to cover it with margarine. Cover with a cloth and set in a warm place until doubled in volume.

Use 1½ teaspoons margarine to grease the sides and bottom of a 9" × 13" cake pan. Set aside for later use.

Stir together brown sugar substitute and cinnamon to mix well and set aside for later use.

Turn dough out onto a lightly floured working surface. Knead lightly and form into a ball. Cover with a cloth and let rest for 10 minutes. Roll dough out to form about a 9" × 16" rectangle. Spread the softened 1½ table-spoons of margarine evenly over the dough. Sprinkle evenly with the sugar substitute and cinnamon mixture. Roll into a long roll like a jelly roll and cut into 24 equal slices. Place the slices, cut side down, in the cake pan, spacing them evenly. Cover with a cloth and let rise until doubled in volume. Bake at 375° F. for 25–30 minutes, or until golden brown. Turn rolls out of the pan onto a wire rack and serve warm, if possible. Serve 1 roll per serving.

Nutritive values per serving:	CAL	CHO (gm)	PRO (gm)	FAT (gm)	NA (mg)
	99	14	2	4	107

Food exchanges per serving: 1 bread, ½ fat
Low-sodium diets: Omit salt. Use salt-free margarine.

OAT BRAN PANCAKES

Yields 7 pancakes—7 servings

½ **cup all-purpose flour**
½ **cup oat bran**
2 **tablespoons sugar**
½ **teaspoon soda**
¼ **teaspoon salt**
¼ **cup dry buttermilk**
1 **cup water at room temperature**
2 **large egg whites or** ¼ **cup liquid egg substitute**
2 **tablespoons vegetable oil**

Place flour, oat bran, sugar, soda, salt, and dry buttermilk in mixer bowl and mix well at low speed. Beat water, egg whites or liquid egg substitute, and oil together with a fork to blend well. Add to flour mixture and beat until almost smooth.

Lightly grease a griddle and preheat to 375° F. (the fat on the griddle has been included in your fat exchange). Pour ⅓ cup batter onto griddle and cook about 3 minutes on one side, or until bubbles begin to form on surface and edges of pancake are dry. Turn and cook 2–3 minutes on other side, or until nicely browned. Repeat with remaining batter and serve hot using 1 pancake per serving.

Nutritive values per serving:	CAL	CHO (gm)	PRO (gm)	FAT (gm)	NA (mg)
	100	15	3	4	165

Food exchanges per serving: 1 bread, 1 fat
Low-sodium diets: Omit salt.

NOODLES

I call this noodle *dough, the Italians call it* pasta, *and the Polish call it* kluski. *It can be cut wide for lasagna, square for manicotti, thin and narrow for fettucini, or in small squares for some types of southern noodles. I also use it for ravioli or cut it thin and narrow to use with spaghetti sauce.*

Remember, when you're deciding which noodles to use, keep in mind that oat bran noodles are very chewy, and wheat noodles have a nutty taste.

Ingredients	Basic	Oat Bran	Wheat
Bread flour	2¼ cups	2 cups	1 cup
Oat bran cereal	none	1 cup	none
Whole wheat flour	none	none	1 cup
Salt	1 teaspoon for all recipes		
Liquid egg substitute	¾ cup	½ cup	½ cup
Lukewarm water	¼ cup	½ cup	½ cup
Vegetable oil	1 tablespoon for all recipes		
Yellow food coloring	2 drops	2 drops	none
Raw yield	20 ounces	24 ounces	20 ounces
Cooked yield	10 cups	12 cups	10 cups

Place dry ingredients in mixer bowl and mix at low speed for ½ minute to blend well. Beat liquid ingredients together with a fork to blend well. Add to dry ingredients and beat, using dough hook, at medium speed for 4 minutes. Turn out onto lightly floured working surface and knead a few times. Form into a ball, place on lightly floured working surface, cover with a cloth, and let stand for 30 minutes to 1 hour.

Divide dough into 3 equal portions. Work with 1 portion at a time, keeping the other 2 portions covered with the cloth. Roll each portion into a very thin rectangle (I like to use my marble rolling pin) on a floured surface. As you roll out the dough, lightly sprinkle the surface with flour to keep it from sticking to the rolling pin. The dough can be cut immediately with a noodle cutter or allowed to dry flat for about 1 hour and then rolled up like a jelly roll and cut with a sharp knife into noodles as wide as you like. You can also use a noodle machine, as I do, for more uniform noodles. Shake out the strips and lay them on a lightly floured towel if you are not going to use them immediately. If the room is sufficiently warm and dry, they should dry in a few hours or overnight; then they can be used right away or stored in the freezer or an airtight container until you need them.

Noodles can also be frozen without drying first. Spread a layer of noodles on a piece of waxed paper, sprinkle with a little flour, and repeat, stacking layers of waxed paper and noodles on top of one another. Wrap the layers in an airtight package and freeze until needed. *Do not defrost noodles before you use them.* Just drop into boiling liquid, as you would fresh noodles, stir until separated, and cook about 20 minutes, or until tender.

When you are ready to cook the noodles, drop them into boiling water or broth, add 1 tablespoon vegetable oil to the pot, and simmer for 10–20 minutes depending on the thickness of the noodles. Drain well. Toss with a little margarine and serve hot, or prepare as directed by recipe in which you are using them.

NUTRITIVE VALUES PER CUP OF COOKED NOODLES

Values	Basic	Oat Bran	Wheat
Calories	126	108	108
CHO (gm)	18	20	16
PRO (gm)	6	6	3
FAT (gm)	4	2	2
Sodium (mg)	236	192	228
Serving for 1 bread exchange	1 cup	¾ cup	1 cup
Meat exchange per serving	1	1	0

Low-sodium diets: Omit salt.

CINNAMON SPREAD

Yields 1 cup—24 servings

This counts as a regular fat exchange but it adds something special to toast or hot breads. I keep some in the refrigerator most of the time and I have given it, in a pretty little ceramic pot, to other diabetics for Christmas or birthday presents. You can vary it using other spices but I prefer cinnamon.

8 ounces soft margarine at room temperature
2 teaspoons ground cinnamon
Granulated sugar substitute equal to ½ cup sugar

Combine ingredients and mix well. Return to container and refrigerate except when it is being used. Yields 24 servings of 1 teaspoon each.

Nutritive values per serving:	CAL	CHO (gm)	PRO (gm)	FAT (gm)	NA (mg)
	34	0	0	4	47

Food exchanges per serving: 1 fat
Low-sodium diets: Use salt-free margarine.

CINNAMON SHAKE

Yields ½ cup

This is good to shake on hot buttered toast, cereal, baked apples, or other fruit, or as directed in recipes in this book.

Granulated sugar substitute equal to ½ cup sugar
1 teaspoon ground cinnamon

Mix sugar substitute and cinnamon well. Put in a shaker and use as desired.

Nutritive values per serving: May be used as desired without adding any nutritive values.

Food exchanges per serving: None
Low-sodium diets: May be used as written.

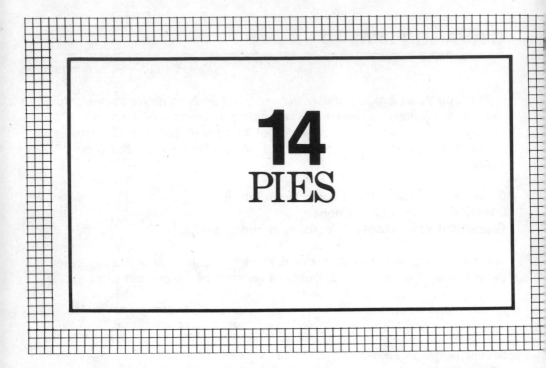

14
PIES

Man lives not by bread alone. Most people want an occasional piece of pie along with their bread, and if we have to give up some bread to have our pie, well, isn't it worth it once in awhile? I, for one, think it is better to enjoy a small piece of pie occasionally and know I can have it once in awhile than to feel deprived and think I'll never be able to eat pie again.

It isn't advisable to buy already prepared pie, even if it is advertised as low calorie, because you don't know what kind of fat is used in the crust and filling—and this is very important on a low-cholesterol diet. It is best to make the crust and filling at home and then you will know it is prepared correctly.

It is difficult to make a good crust without a certain amount of fat. We can cut the fat back a little bit, but it still requires a fair amount of fat to have a tender crust. Since the crust is necessarily high in fat and calories, it is better to serve one-crust pies rather than double-crust pies and to use a filling that is lower in calories.

The pie crust recipes in this chapter yield just enough dough for a single crust. If you want to make a double-crust pie, double the recipe and it will be the correct amount of dough for a double crust. It won't be enough for the elaborate edges and fancy decorations that some good cooks like to add to their pies, but it will be enough for a generous crust.

If you want to make a pie filling using your own recipe, you can calculate the exchanges for the filling according to Chapter 2 and then use it in one of the crusts in this chapter. Sometimes you may have to work with your filling a little bit to get it down to where you can afford it, but if it is a family favorite it can be worthwhile to work on it.

Of course, we use unsweetened fruits and sugar substitutes routinely, and don't forget that diabetic puddings make good pie fillings. You can use a diabetic pudding and a couple of fresh bananas to make a very good banana pie, and you can always garnish it with a couple of tablespoons of Whipped Topping (see index).

I have included the exchange values of the pie crust in the pie recipes. If you need to know the values of the filling, you can subtract the values of the crust from the total values of the pie.

MOM'S PIE CRUST

Yields 1 9-inch crust—8 servings

This is the crust that my mother always made. She used lard until we started following a low-cholesterol meal pattern; then she changed to margarine. She always said that she couldn't make good pie crust until she started using this recipe—and then she never had a failure.

⅓ **cup (⅔ stick) margarine**
2 tablespoons water
1 cup all-purpose flour
¼ **teaspoon baking powder**
¼ **teaspoon salt**
Warm water

Heat margarine and 2 tablespoons water together until margarine is melted. Set aside to cool to room temperature. Place flour, baking powder, and salt in mixing bowl and stir to blend well. Mix margarine mixture with a fork to blend and then add to flour mixture.

Add warm water by the tablespoonful to crust mixture, if necessary. (It will depend upon the type of flour, but I've never needed to add more than 2 tablespoons to any flour that I have used.) Round dough into a ball and let set, covered, at room temperature for 15–30 minutes. Roll crust out on a lightly floured working surface to form a circle. Fit into 9-inch pie pan and prick the bottom 6 or 7 times with the tines of a fork. Bake at 425° F. for 12–15 minutes or until lightly browned. Cool and fill with desired filling; or fill the unbaked crust with desired filling and bake according to directions with the filling.

I use two pie pans when I'm making a single crust. I place the crust in the bottom pan, prick it with a fork, and then put another pan exactly the same size on top of the crust, and bake it about 15 minutes or until lightly browned. I then remove it from the oven and remove the top pan, cool to room temperature, and use as desired.

Serve ⅛ of the crust per serving.

Nutritive values per serving:	CAL	CHO (gm)	PRO (gm)	FAT (gm)	NA (mg)
	125	12	2	8	170

Food exchanges per serving: 1 fruit, 1½ fat
Low-sodium diets: Omit salt. Use low-sodium baking powder and salt-free margarine.

SOUTHERN PIE CRUST

Yields 1 9-inch crust—8 servings

This crust isn't as yellow as it is when it is made with egg yolks. If you like the yellow color, you can add a drop or two of yellow coloring to the ice water when you are mixing the crust.

½ cup cake flour
½ cup all-purpose flour
⅓ cup (⅔ stick) margarine from the refrigerator
¼ cup ice water
¼ teaspoon salt
1 egg white
1½ teaspoons white vinegar

Place flours in bowl and stir to blend. Cut margarine into the flour until the mixture resembles coarse meal.

Combine water, salt, egg white, and vinegar in a cup. Mix well with a fork and then add to the flour mixture. Mix lightly with a fork until you can round the pastry into a ball. Refrigerate, or cover and let set at room temperature for 15 to 30 minutes. Roll crust out on a lightly floured working surface to form a circle. Fit into 9-inch pie tin and prick the bottom 6 or 7 times with the tines of a fork. Bake at 425° F. for 12–15 minutes, or until lightly browned. Cool and fill with the desired filling; or fill the unbaked crust with the desired filling and bake according to directions with the filling. Serve ⅛ of the pie per portion.

Nutritive values per serving:	CAL	CHO (gm)	PRO (gm)	FAT (gm)	NA (mg)
	124	12	2	8	163

Food exchanges per serving: 1 fruit, 1½ fat
Low-sodium diets: Omit salt. Use salt-free margarine.

GRAHAM CRACKER CRUST

Yields 1 9-inch crust—8 servings

I like to bake this crust because that makes it crisp. If you want a softer crust, refrigerate it after it is prepared instead of baking it.

8 crushed graham crackers (2½-inch squares)
3 tablespoons melted margarine
2 tablespoons sugar

Combine ingredients in 9-inch pie tin and mix well with your fingers. Press crumbs evenly around the edges and on the bottom of the pie tin. Bake at 350° F. for 6 minutes. Cool and fill as desired. Cut into 8 even portions, using 1 portion per serving.

Nutritive values per serving:	CAL	CHO (gm)	PRO (gm)	FAT (gm)	NA (mg)
	78	8	1	5	100

Food exchanges per serving: ½ bread, 1 fat
Low-sodium diets: Use salt-free margarine.

APPLE PIE

Yields 1 9-inch pie—8 servings

FILLING
7 tart medium (4 to the pound) apples
¾ cup Brown Sugar Twin
2 tablespoons flour
⅛ teaspoon nutmeg or mace
1 teaspoon cinnamon
¼ teaspoon salt

Crust for 2-crust pie (see index)
2 tablespoons margarine

Peel and core apples and slice thinly. Stir together Sugar Twin, flour, nutmeg, cinnamon, and salt to blend and then mix lightly with apples.

Fill bottom crust evenly with apple mixture. Dot with margarine. Cut slits in upper crust and place over filling. Seal pie crust at the edges and bake at 400° F. for 50 minutes, or until pie is browned and well done. Cool to room temperature on wire rack. Cut into 8 equal pieces and serve 1 piece per serving.

Nutritive values per serving (including double crust):	CAL	CHO (gm)	PRO (gm)	FAT (gm)	NA (mg)
	336	39	3	19	443

Food exchanges per serving: 2 bread, ½ fruit, 4 fat
Low-sodium diets: Omit salt. Use salt-free margarine and low-sodium pie crust.

CHERRY PIE

Yields 1 9-inch pie—8 servings

This is my husband's favorite pie. He always looks for it when we go to church dinners in this area because the women who live here in Iowa are such wonderful cooks and their pies are fabulous. In the fall it seems as though we go to a church dinner at least once a week—and all of them are good.

FILLING
2 16-ounce cans unsweetened red cherries
1 cup liquid from the cherries
1 tablespoon cornstarch
¼ teaspoon almond flavoring
Sugar substitute equal to 1 cup sugar

1 prebaked single pie crust (see index)
Whipped Topping (see index)

Drain cherries well, reserving 1 cup liquid. Set cherries aside and combine 1 cup liquid and cornstarch. Cook and stir over moderate heat until thickened and transparent and the starchy taste is gone. Remove from heat and add sugar substitute, almond flavoring, and cherries. Taste and add more sweetener, if desired. Cool to room temperature.

Spread filling evenly in crust. Let set at least 15 minutes. Cut into 8 equal portions and serve 1 portion per serving. Garnish each serving of pie with 1 or 2 tablespoons Whipped Topping, if desired.

Nutritive values per portion (including crust):	CAL	CHO (gm)	PRO (gm)	FAT (gm)	NA (mg)
	177	25	3	8	173
Food exchanges per serving:	1 bread, ½ fruit, 2 fat				
Low-sodium diets:	Use salt-free pie crust.				

CUSTARD PIE

Yields 1 9-inch pie—8 servings

This recipe is from Vera Wilson, a friend of mine here in Wadena. Vera has been a great help to me in writing this book—she not only gave me several recipes, but she also listened to me when I was troubled over parts of the book and rejoiced with me when everything came out okay.

FILLING
1 cup liquid egg substitute
2 tablespoons sugar
Sugar substitute equal to ⅓ cup sugar
1 teaspoon vanilla
¼ teaspoon salt
1 teaspoon cornstarch
¾ cup instant dry milk
2 cups water

1 unbaked crust (see index)
Ground nutmeg as desired

Combine all filling ingredients and mix thoroughly. Pour filling into unbaked pie crust.

Sprinkle nutmeg over filling and bake at 475° F. for 10 minutes. Reduce heat to 425° F. without opening the oven door and bake another 15 minutes. Test to see if it is done by sticking a knife in the center of the pie—if the knife doesn't come out clean, bake another 5 minutes. (It has always been done for me at the end of 15 minutes but Vera said to be sure and include that caution.) Cool to room temperature out of drafts. Cut into 8 pieces and serve 1 piece per serving.

Nutritive values per serving (including crust):	CAL	CHO (gm)	PRO (gm)	FAT (gm)	NA (mg)
	186	18	7	10	308

Food exchanges per serving: 1 milk, 1 vegetable, 2 fat
Low-sodium diets: Omit salt. Use salt-free pie crust.

KEY LIME PIE

Yields 1 9-inch pie—8 servings

When I was in Key West with Bud and Frances Gunsallus, she ordered Key Lime Pie and gave me a bite of it. It was delicious and I decided I'd like to be able to make it for myself. Fortunately for me, Searle's published a recipe for it in one of their advertisements and I was quick to try it and serve it back here in Iowa. You can make it with lemon juice, but it is the lime juice which makes it authentic.

FILLING
1 packet Knox Unflavored Gelatine
3 tablespoons lime juice
½ cup boiling water
9 1-gram packets Equal (aspartame) sugar substitute
1 cup evaporated skim milk
1 teaspoon vanilla
Juice of 1½ limes
2 drops green food coloring

1 9-inch graham cracker crust (see index)
Lime zest
Thin lime slices

Sprinkle gelatin over lime juice and let it stand for 1 minute. Add boiling water and sweetener to gelatin mixture and stir until gelatin is dissolved. Refrigerate about 45 minutes or until slightly thickened.

Combine milk and vanilla and freeze 30 minutes. Remove from freezer and whip at high speed until stiff. Stir lime juice and food coloring into whipped milk. (Save remaining ½ lime for garnish.) Slowly blend gelatin mixture into whipped milk.

Spoon pie filling into crust. Chill until firm. Garnish with lime zest and lime slices. Cut into 8 even portions and serve 1 portion per serving.

Nutritive values per serving (including crust):	CAL	CHO (gm)	PRO (gm)	FAT (gm)	NA (mg)
	111	14	4	5	132

Food exchanges per serving: 1 bread, 1 fat
Low-sodium diets: Use salt-free crust.

LEMON PIE

Yields 1 9-inch pie—8 servings

FILLING
2 large egg whites at room temperature
¼ teaspoon cream of tartar
¼ cup sugar
1 cup water
3 tablespoons lemon juice
2 tablespoons cornstarch
Grated rind of 1 lemon
1 tablespoon margarine
3 drops yellow food coloring
8 1-gram packets Equal (aspartame)

1 9-inch graham cracker crust (see index)

Beat egg whites until frothy. Add cream of tartar and continue to beat at high speed, gradually adding sugar until meringue is stiff.

Combine water, lemon juice, and cornstarch in a small saucepan and stir until smooth. Add lemon rind, margarine, and food coloring to cornstarch mixture and cook and stir over moderate heat until thickened and the starchy taste is gone. Remove from heat. Mix sweetener into hot cooked mixture. Fold hot cooked mixture into meringue and mix lightly but thoroughly.

Pour filling into crust and refrigerate until firm. Cut into 8 equal pieces and serve 1 piece per serving.

Nutritive values per serving (including graham cracker crust):	CAL	CHO (gm)	PRO (gm)	FAT (gm)	NA (mg)
	132	18	2	6	130
Food exchanges per serving:	1 bread, 1 fat				
Low-sodium diets:	Use salt-free margarine and salt-free pie crust.				

PUMPKIN PIE

Yields 1 9-inch pie—8 servings

Every year when we have our annual church dinner in the fall, Cecile Moats and I cut and serve the pies, and it keeps both of us busy. We have noticed that pumpkin and sour cream raisin pies are the most popular, with cherry and apple right behind them. I've really tried, but I can't manage a sour cream raisin pie that fits into our diets—but we can have pumpkin, apple, and cherry, so let's enjoy them!

FILLING
1 16-ounce can solid-pack pumpkin
½ cup liquid egg substitute
2 tablespoons sugar
Sugar substitute equal to ⅓ cup sugar
½ teaspoon salt
2 teaspoons pumpkin pie spice
1⅔ cups water
½ cup instant dry milk

1 unbaked 9-inch pie crust (see index)

Combine filling ingredients and mix until smooth.

Pour filling into the unbaked pie crust. Be careful to build up the crust around the edges of the pan because the pie will puff while it is baking. Bake at 425° F. for 15 minutes. Reduce the temperature of the oven to 350° F. without opening the oven door and continue to bake for another 45 minutes, or until a knife inserted in the center of the pie comes out clean. Cool to room temperature. Cut into 8 even portions and serve 1 piece per serving.

Nutritive values per serving (including crust):	CAL	CHO (gm)	PRO (gm)	FAT (gm)	NA (mg)
	184	22	5	9	338

Food exchanges per serving: 1 bread, ½ fruit, ½ lean meat, 1 fat
Low-sodium diets: Omit salt. Use salt-free pie crust.

PUMPKIN SCOTCH PIE

Yields 1 9-inch pie—8 servings

This recipe is from Dorothea Odekirk of Fayette, Iowa. Dorothea and I both belong to the Fayette County Branch of the American Association of University Women and she gave me this recipe after I had talked about my new book one night at a meeting. She prepares this for her husband, who is diabetic.

FILLING
1 2⅛ ounce package D-Zerta low-calorie butterscotch pudding
1¾ cups skim milk
1 cup precooked canned pumpkin
¼ cup Brown Sugar Twin sugar substitute
1 teaspoon pumpkin pie spice

1 9-inch graham cracker crust (see index)
Whipped Topping (see index)

Empty package of pudding mix into small saucepan. Add milk gradually. Cook and stir over moderate heat until pudding comes to a boil. Remove from heat. Add pumpkin, sweetener, and spice to cooked pudding. Mix well.

Pour filling into prepared crust. Refrigerate until served. Cut into 8 equal portions and serve 1 portion per serving. Garnish with whipped topping just before pie is served, if desired (2 tablespoons topping is free).

Nutritive values per serving (including crust):	CAL	CHO (gm)	PRO (gm)	FAT (gm)	NA (mg)
	122	17	3	5	168

Food exchanges per serving: 1 bread, 1 fat
Low-sodium diets: Use salt-free crust.

STRAWBERRY CHIFFON PIE

Yields 1 9-inch pie—8 servings

This pie is pretty enough to serve for a ladies' luncheon and it is as good as it looks. You can use different flavors of soft drink mix if you like, with different garnishes.

FILLING
1 cup water
1 envelope Knox Unflavored Gelatine
1 .20-ounce packet Wyler's unsweetened flavored soft drink mix or Kool-Aid unsweetened soft drink mix
8 1-gram packets Equal (aspartame) sugar substitute
1 recipe Whipped Topping (see index)
2 tablespoons instant dry milk

9-inch graham cracker crust (see index)
9 fresh strawberries (optional)

Combine water and gelatin. Let set for 5 minutes and then heat until gelatin is melted. Add soft drink mix and sweetener to gelatin. Mix well and refrigerate until slightly thickened.

Prepare Whipped Topping while gelatin is thickening. Refrigerate until needed. Add dry milk to thickened gelatin and whip at high speed until creamy and stiff. Remove beater and gently fold whipped topping into whipped gelatin.

Spread filling evenly in graham cracker crust. Garnish each serving with a fresh strawberry, placing a fresh strawberry in the center of the pie. Refrigerate until firm. Cut into 8 equal pieces and serve 1 piece per serving.

Nutritive values per serving (including crust and topping):	CAL	CHO (gm)	PRO (gm)	FAT (gm)	NA (mg)
	125	15	3	7	122
Food exchanges per serving:	1 bread, 1 fat				
Low-sodium diets:	Use salt-free crust.				

WHIPPED TOPPING

Yields 3 cups topping—24 servings

This topping may be spread on top of a pie or used as a garnish for pies, puddings, or gelatins. It should be prepared as close to serving time as possible since it loses volume after a period of time.

½ cup instant dry milk
⅓ cup cold water
2 tablespoons lemon juice
2 tablespoons sugar
Dry sugar substitute equal to ¼ cup sugar (optional)
½ teaspoon vanilla

Combine dry milk and water and refrigerate for 30 minutes. Beat at high speed for 4 minutes.

Add lemon juice to whipped milk and beat at high speed for 4 minutes. Stir the sugar and sugar substitute together and add gradually to the whipped milk while it is being beaten. Add vanilla to whipped topping and refrigerate until used. Yields 24 servings of 2 tablespoons each.

Nutritive values per serving:	CAL	CHO (gm)	PRO (gm)	FAT (gm)	NA (mg)
	12	2	negl.	negl.	6

Food exchanges per serving: 2 tablespoons may be considered free (⅓ cup is 1 vegetable exchange)

Low-sodium diets: May be used as written.

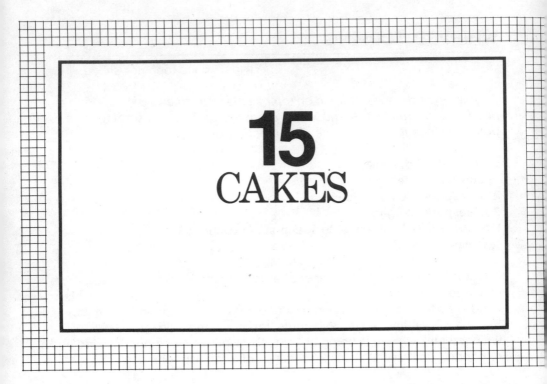

15
CAKES

Most diabetics long for the cakes and cookies that we used to enjoy so much. In fact, when I asked my friends and other diabetics what recipes they would like to see in this book, most of them started out with, "Some really good cakes and cookies." That is a tough request for a diabetic cookbook and gets even tougher when the recipes also need to be suitable for a low-cholesterol diet.

We all know that we can't have cake and cookies for every meal, because we need to save the exchanges for more important foods—but there are times such as birthdays when you really would like to be able to eat a piece of cake along with everyone else. Another time I like to have diabetic cake or cookies on hand is when we have unexpected guests and I want to offer them cake or cookies along with their coffee or tea. This is a great area for coffee and a sweet, but until I started to make my own cake or cookies, I always just sat there and sipped coffee. Now I can have something with it and I'm much happier and more relaxed when we have guests. I also have learned to slip a couple of my diabetic cookies in my purse (well-wrapped, of course) and take them along with me when we are invited out for afternoon coffee. Hostesses don't seem to mind so much if I eat my own cookies as long as I have something.

Let's face it. We will probably never get a really fine-textured cake suitable for a diabetic diet because the percentage of sugar in a cake is very important to the texture of the cake. However, we can get an acceptable cake if we use ingredients at room temperature and follow the directions for making the cake very carefully, using the recipes that follow.

A cake suitable for a low-cholesterol diet needs to avoid whole eggs, butter, cream, lard, and whole milk. Therefore, a cake suitable for a low-cholesterol diabetic diet needs to be made with margarine or oil, egg whites or liquid egg substitute, fat-free milk, and last but not least, very little sugar or other sweetener. I'm sorry to say that I haven't been able to make sponge cake, jelly roll, genoise, or those lovely Hungarian tortes with the liquid egg substitute. I've tried, but for me it remains an impossible dream.

I have managed to develop some cakes suitable for the low-cholesterol diabetic diet using approved ingredients which I think you will like. I found that cocoa used with buttermilk and baking soda gives a good texture. I also managed to develop several other good cakes, including some with syrup or molasses. I used the regular corn syrup, but you can use fructose syrup if you like sweeter cakes. I did use a little sugar or syrup, which I counted when I analyzed the recipes. You might discuss the use of either with your doctor before preparing these recipes, but since both are part of the carbohydrate allowance, most doctors feel that it is permissible to use them.

Instant dry milk and dry buttermilk are used in many of these recipes because I find them so convenient. They are generally lower in cost than the fresh skim milk or buttermilk made with skim milk and they can be kept unopened on the shelf or in the refrigerator after they are opened, if you like, for a fairly long period of time. It isn't all that easy in our area to get fresh buttermilk made with skim milk and for that reason also I like to keep the powdered buttermilk on hand. It is nationally available so if your store doesn't carry it, I'm sure they can get it for you.

Technique, or the way you mix the cake, is very important when you are making a cake, and even more so when you are working with very little sugar. Because of the high proportion of flour to sugar, it is easy to mix the flour too much, which develops the gluten in the flour. That is all to the good when you are making bread, but can be a disaster when you are making a cake. When the gluten in the cake has been developed too much, you get a very tough cake with large air holes. Therefore, it is important to cream the fat and the little bit of sugar very well—but to add the flour mixture very carefully and mix it only as much as is absolutely necessary.

I hope that you will use these recipes as a basis for your own needs. Add fruit to them for a shortcake, garnish them with a couple of tablespoons of

Whipped Topping (see index), layer them with diabetic jelly between the layers, and sprinkle them with Sugar Twin instead of powdered sugar—or add various flavorings to the cakes to vary their flavor. They can be the basis for lots of interesting desserts.

I have used a minimum of sugar substitute in these recipes because that is how we prefer them. If you want an increased amount, feel free to vary the amount according to your own tastes; it won't affect the final recipe if used within normal bounds. I have also shown the amount according to the sugar equivalents because that is how people tell me they prefer to have recipes written.

Of course, when you are making low-cholesterol diabetic cake, you need to follow all of the suggestions for a good cake made with the ordinary amount of sugar:

1. Have all ingredients at room temperature unless the directions state otherwise. This is particularly important for the liquid egg substitute. Don't use it right from the refrigerator in a cake or cookie.

2. Use stick margarine unless the recipe specifies soft margarine.

3. Always read the recipe thoroughly before you start to prepare it to be sure that you understand it and that you have all of the ingredients on hand. I like to get out all of the ingredients and prepare the pans before I start mixing the cake. These recipes also presume that the oven will be pre-heated, so I generally start the oven also when I start to mix the cake.

4. Always use regulation-size measuring cups and spoons and bake cakes in the size pan specified in the recipe. An otherwise good cake can be ruined if baked in the wrong size pan. If you want to bake a cake in a smaller pan, fill the pan ⅔ full of batter and bake any remaining batter as cupcakes.

5. Don't sift the flour unless the recipe directs you to do so. Sifting changes the amount of flour in a cup. I never sift flour. I always combine the ingredients and stir them together. This is much simpler and yields the same results.

6. Follow the recipe exactly the first time. Then you can change it if you like after you are sure that you want to make a change in it. Don't forget that if you add nuts or raisins or other goodies to a recipe, you need to count those added ingredients in your diet.

7. Use margarine, not oil, to grease your pans. I like to use the margarine wrapper with a little bit of the margarine left on it to grease the pan for a cake that includes margarine as an ingredient.

8. These cakes were all tested in metal pans. If you use a glass baking dish, decrease the baking temperature 25° F.

9. When you want to defrost a cake that has been frozen, it should be unwrapped and placed in a refrigerator until it is defrosted. If you try to defrost it at room temperature in the wrappings it will get sticky, and if you defrost it unwrapped at room temperature it will collect moisture and be soggy. I always had a rough time trying to get a cake defrosted without ruining it until Thelma Richburg of Columbia, South Carolina, told me how to do it successfully, and it really works this way. She is the mother of Olivia Sniffin, one of my favorite cousins-in-law. Mrs. Richburg bakes a lot of cakes and decorates them for special occasions and really knows how to bake good cakes—and how to take care of them after they are baked.

COCOA CAKE

Yields 1 2-layer cake—16 servings

This recipe is based on one from Lois Erickson who lives in the country near Wadena. Lois has a way with roses and brought several wild roses for me to plant because I felt we should have some of Iowa's state flower in our backyard.

½ **cup cocoa**
½ **cup boiling water**
¾ **cup (1½ sticks) margarine at room temperature**
Liquid sugar substitute equal to ½ cup sugar
2 teaspoons vanilla
3 large egg whites at room temperature
½ **teaspoon cream of tartar**
⅓ **cup sugar**
2½ **cups cake flour**
1 teaspoon baking soda
2 teaspoons baking powder
¼ **teaspoon salt**
½ **teaspoon cinnamon**
1 cup cool water

Mix together cocoa and boiling water to blend and set aside to cool to room temperature. Cream margarine at medium speed until light and fluffy. Add sweetener and vanilla to creamed mixture, along with cooled cocoa mixture. Mix at medium speed until well blended.

Beat egg whites at medium speed until foamy. Add cream of tartar and beat at high speed, gradually adding sugar, to form a meringue. Set aside for later use. Stir together flour, soda, baking powder, salt, and cinnamon to blend well.

Add 1 cup water to creamed mixture along with flour mixture. Beat at medium speed for 1–2 minutes or until well blended. Stir batter carefully into the meringue. Spread ½ of the batter evenly in each of 2 9-inch cake layer pans that have been greased with margarine and lined on the bottom with wax paper. Bake at 350° F. for 30–35 minutes, or until a cake tester comes out clean from the center of the cake and the cake pulls away from the sides of the pan. Turn cake out onto a cake cooler, remove the paper, and cool to room temperature.

Put diabetic jelly between the cake layers and frost at the last minute with

Fluffy Frosting (see index). Cut cake into 16 equal servings.

Nutritive values per serving:	CAL	CHO (gm)	PRO (gm)	FAT (gm)	NA (mg)
	170	20	3	9	263

Food exchanges per serving: 1⅓ bread, 2 fat
Low-sodium diets: Omit salt. Use salt-free margarine and low-sodium baking powder.

CHOCOLATE CAKE

Yields 1 cake—16 servings

¾ cup (1½ sticks) margarine at room temperature
¼ cup sugar
½ cup liquid egg substitute at room temperature
Liquid sugar substitute equal to ⅓ cup sugar
2 teaspoons vanilla
2 cups cake flour
2 teaspoons baking powder
¼ cup instant dry milk
⅓ cup cocoa
1 cup water at room temperature

Cream together margarine and sugar at medium speed until light and fluffy. Add egg substitute, sweetener, and vanilla to creamed mixture and beat at medium speed for ½ minute.

Stir together flour, baking powder, dry milk, and cocoa to blend.

Add 1 cup water to creamed mixture along with flour mixture and mix at medium speed only until smooth. Spread evenly in a 9-inch square pan that has been greased with margarine. Bake at 350° F. for 30–35 minutes, or until a cake tester comes out clean and the cake pulls away from the sides of the pan. Cool to room temperature and cut 4 × 4 to yield 16 equal servings.

Nutritive values per serving:	CAL	CHO (gm)	PRO (gm)	FAT (gm)	NA (mg)
	157	16	3	9	175

Food exchanges per serving: 1 bread, 2 fat
Low-sodium diets: Use salt-free margarine and low-sodium baking powder.

DEVIL'S FOOD CAKE

Yields 1 cake—18 servings

½ **cup cocoa**
½ **cup boiling water**
2 **cups cake flour**
½ **teaspoon baking soda**
1½ **teaspoons baking powder**
⅛ **teaspoon salt**
⅓ **cup sugar**
¾ **cup liquid egg substitute at room temperature**
Liquid sugar substitute equal to ¾ cup sugar
1 **teaspoon vanilla**
½ **cup (1 stick) margarine at room temperature**

Stir together cocoa and boiling water until smooth. Set aside to cool to room temperature.

Place flour, soda, baking powder, salt, and sugar in mixer bowl and mix at low speed about 1 minute to blend.

Add egg substitute, sweetener, and vanilla to cocoa mixture and mix well.

Add margarine to dry ingredients along with cocoa mixture and mix at medium speed about 1 minute or until well blended. Pour into a 9-inch square or 9" × 13" cake pan that has been greased with margarine. Bake at 350° F. for about 30 minutes, or until a cake tester comes out clean and the cake pulls away from the sides of the pan. Cool in the pan and cut 6 × 3 to yield 18 pieces. Serve cold with a tablespoon of Whipped Topping (see index) or warm with some Chocolate Sauce (see index). Allow 1 piece per serving.

Nutritive values per serving without topping:	CAL	CHO (gm)	PRO (gm)	FAT (gm)	NA (mg)
	119	16	2	6	210
Food exchanges per serving:	1 bread, 1 fat				

Low-sodium diets: Omit salt. Use low-sodium baking powder and salt-free margarine.

OATMEAL CAKE

Yields 1 cake—16 servings

This cake recipe from Thelma VanLaningham of Independence, Iowa, provides some fiber in the oatmeal and raisins. It is mildly spiced with an old-fashioned flavor.

1 cup all-purpose flour
1 teaspoon baking soda
½ teaspoon salt
1 teaspoon cinnamon
½ teaspoon nutmeg
⅓ cup dry buttermilk
¼ cup (½ stick) margarine at room temperature
3 large egg whites at room temperature
¼ cup dark molasses
Liquid sugar substitute equal to 3 tablespoons sugar
¾ cup water at room temperature, divided
1 cup rolled oats
¼ cup raisins

Place flour, soda, salt, cinnamon, nutmeg, and dry buttermilk in mixer bowl and mix at low speed to blend. Add margarine, egg whites, molasses, sweetener, and ½ cup water to flour mixture and beat at medium speed for 1 minute to mix well.

Add ¼ cup water, oats, and raisins to batter and mix at medium speed only until blended. Spread batter evenly in a 9-inch square pan that has been greased with margarine. Bake at 375° F. for about 30 minutes, or until a cake tester comes out clean and the cake pulls away from the sides of the pan. Cut cake 4 × 4 into 16 equal servings.

Nutritive values per serving:

	CAL	CHO (gm)	PRO (gm)	FAT (gm)	NA (mg)
	104	14	3	3	194

Food exchanges per serving: 1 bread, ½ fat
Low-sodium diets: Omit salt. Use salt-free margarine.

RAISIN CAKE

Yields 1 cake—20 servings

This cake from Ruth Schoephoerster of Oelwein, Iowa, tastes like the fruit cake my mother used to make when I was a child. Ruth belongs to the Hub City Chapter of the Iowa Affiliate of the American Diabetes Association, to which I also belong, and I see her there often at meetings.

1 cup raisins
Boiling water as necessary
Liquid sugar substitute equal to ¾ cup sugar
3 large egg whites
½ cup oil
1½ teaspoons vanilla
1 cup unsweetened applesauce
2 cups all-purpose flour
1 teaspoon baking soda
1 teaspoon baking powder
1¼ teaspoons cinnamon
½ teaspoon nutmeg
½ teaspoon salt

Cover raisins with water. Let stand 5 minutes. Drain well and place the raisins in a mixer bowl. Discard the liquid. Add sweetener, egg whites, oil, vanilla, and applesauce to raisins and mix at medium speed for a few seconds to blend.

Blend remaining dry ingredients well and add to raisin mixture. Mix at medium speed to blend. Spread evenly in a 9″ × 13″ cake pan that has been greased with margarine. Bake at 350° F. for 35–40 minutes, or until well browned and the cake has drawn away from the sides of the pan. Cut 4 × 5 to yield 20 pieces. Serve 1 piece per serving.

Nutritive values per serving:	CAL	CHO (gm)	PRO (gm)	FAT (gm)	NA (mg)
	122	17	2	6	131

Food exchanges per serving: 1 bread, 1 fat
Low-sodium diets: Omit salt. Use low-sodium baking powder.

SPICE CUPCAKES

Yields 9 cupcakes—9 servings

2 cups cake flour
⅓ cup brown sugar
1 teaspoon cinnamon
1½ teaspoons baking powder
½ cup water at room temperature
Liquid sugar substitute equal to ⅓ cup sugar
½ cup liquid egg substitute at room temperature
⅓ cup vegetable oil
2 teaspoons vanilla

Place flour, sugar, cinnamon, and baking powder in mixer bowl and mix at low speed to blend well.

Mix together ½ cup water, sweetener, egg substitute, oil, and vanilla with a fork. Add to flour mixture and mix with a spoon only until well blended. Grease 9 muffin tins with margarine or line with paper. Fill muffin tins about ½ full and bake at 375° F. for 20–25 minutes, or until well browned. Serve 1 cupcake per serving.

Nutritive values per serving:	CAL	CHO (gm)	PRO (gm)	FAT (gm)	NA (mg)
	205	29	3	8	78

Food exchanges per serving: 2 bread, 1½ fat
Low-sodium diets: Use low-sodium baking powder.

WACKY CUPCAKES

Yields 12 cupcakes—12 servings

My sister has been making this cake ever since she was a little girl. The original recipe said to put the dry ingredients in the pan and then add the rest and mix it in the pan you bake it in, but I like this way better.

1½ cups cake flour
¼ cup sugar
¼ cup cocoa
1 teaspoon baking soda
½ teaspoon salt
1 cup water at room temperature
Liquid sugar substitute equal to ½ cup sugar
1 tablespoon vinegar
2 teaspoons vanilla
½ cup vegetable oil

Place flour, sugar, cocoa, soda, and salt in mixer bowl and mix at low speed to blend.

Beat together remaining ingredients with a fork to blend. Add all at once to dry ingredients and beat at medium speed until smooth. Paper-line 12 muffin tins or grease with margarine and flour. Fill muffin tins about ½ full and bake at 350° F. for about 30 minutes, or until a cake tester comes out clean from the center of the cupcake. Serve 1 cupcake per serving.

	CAL	CHO (gm)	PRO (gm)	FAT (gm)	NA (mg)
Nutritive values per serving:	158	17	2	10	188

Food exchanges per serving: 1 bread, 2 fat
Low-sodium diets: Omit salt.

WHITE CAKE

Yields 1 cake—16 servings

This recipe is based on one from Margaret Foxwell of Elgin, Iowa. It has the texture of a firm European cake.

½ **cup (1 stick) margarine at room temperature**
¼ **cup white corn syrup**
Liquid sugar substitute equal to ⅓ cup sugar
2 teaspoons vanilla
3 large egg whites at room temperature
2 cups cake flour
1 tablespoon baking powder
2 tablespoons non-fat dry milk
½ **cup water at room temperature**

Beat margarine, corn syrup, sweetener, vanilla, and egg whites at medium speed about 1 minute or until blended.

Stir together flour, baking powder, and dry milk until well blended.

Add flour mixture and ½ cup water to creamed mixture and stir with a large spoon until well mixed. Do not overbeat. Spread evenly in a 9-inch square pan that has been greased with margarine, and bake at 350° F. for 30–35 minutes or until lightly browned and it pulls away from the sides of the pan. Cool and cut 4 × 4 into 16 equal servings.

Nutritive values per serving:	CAL	CHO (gm)	PRO (gm)	FAT (gm)	NA (mg)
	126	15	2	5	147

Food exchanges per serving: 1 bread, 1 fat
Low-sodium diets: Use salt-free margarine and low-sodium baking powder.

YELLOW CAKE

Yields 1 cake—16 servings

2 cups cake flour
½ teaspoon baking soda
1½ teaspoons baking powder
⅓ cup sugar
3 tablespoons dry buttermilk
¾ cup water at room temperature
⅓ cup vegetable oil
Liquid sugar substitute equal to ¼ cup sugar
2 teaspoons vanilla
½ cup liquid egg substitute at room temperature
¼ cup (½ stick) margarine at room temperature

Place dry ingredients in mixer bowl and mix at low speed to blend well.

Combine ¾ cup water, oil, sweetener, vanilla, and egg substitute and mix with a fork to blend. Add margarine to flour mixture along with liquid mixture and mix with a spoon only until well blended. Spread evenly in a 9-inch square pan which has been greased with margarine. Bake 30–35 minutes at 375° F., or until a cake tester comes out clean and the cake pulls away from the sides of the pan. Cool to room temperature and cut 4 × 4 to yield 16 equal servings.

Nutritive values per serving:	CAL	CHO (gm)	PRO (gm)	FAT (gm)	NA (mg)
	143	17	2	7	119

Food exchanges per serving: 1 bread, 1 fat
Low-sodium diets: Use low-sodium baking powder and salt-free margarine.

FLUFFY FROSTING

Yields about 3 cups frosting—16 servings

This recipe from the makers of Sweet'N Low reminds me of the seven-minute frosting my mother used to make. You can change the frosting easily by adding a couple of drops of food coloring and some flavoring, such as 2 drops of red coloring and some peppermint flavoring.

½ **cup sugar**
2 **tablespoons water**
2 **packets Sweet'N Low**
2 **large egg whites**
¼ **teaspoon cream of tartar**
½ **teaspoon vanilla**

Combine sugar, water, Sweet'N Low, egg whites, and cream of tartar in top of a double boiler and beat at high speed for 1 minute. Set over simmering water in the bottom of the double boiler. Continue to beat at high speed for 4–5 minutes or until soft peaks form. Remove from heat.

Add vanilla to frosting and continue beating at high speed 1–2 minutes or until thick enough to spread on a cooled cake. Use about 2½ tablespoons per portion if frosting individually; or use this amount to frost a 2-layer cake or a 9-inch square cake, both of which would then be cut into 16 equal servings.

Nutritive values per serving:	CAL	CHO (gm)	PRO (gm)	FAT (gm)	NA (mg)
	23	6	negl.	negl.	negl.
Food exchange values per serving:	1 vegetable (1–1½ tablespoons may be used as a topping for cake or pudding without counting it as an exchange)				
Low-sodium diets:	May be used as written.				

LEMON SAUCE

Yields 2 cups—8 servings

This sauce adds a lot to a plain or spice cake—either warm or at room temperature.

2 cups water
2 tablespoons cornstarch
⅛ teaspoon salt
2 tablespoons margarine
2 tablespoons lemon juice
Grated rind of 1 lemon
1 drop yellow food coloring
8 1-gram packets Equal (aspartame) sugar substitute

Combine water, cornstarch, and salt and stir until smooth in a small saucepan. Cook and stir over moderate heat until thickened and clear and then continue to simmer, stirring constantly, for another 2 minutes. Remove from heat.

Add remaining ingredients to sauce and stir lightly to mix well. Serve warm, if possible, over cake or pudding. Serve ¼ cup per serving.

Nutritive values per serving:

	CAL	CHO (gm)	PRO (gm)	FAT (gm)	NA (mg)
	38	3	negl.	3	68

Food exchanges per serving: ½ fat, ½ vegetable
Low-sodium diets: Omit salt. Use salt-free margarine.

CHOCOLATE SAUCE

Yields 1½ cups—12 servings

This is good on ice milk or as a topping for cake or pudding.

3 tablespoons cocoa
4 teaspoons cornstarch
⅓ cup instant dry milk
⅛ teaspoon salt
1½ cups water
1 tablespoon margarine
2 teaspoons vanilla
10 1-gram packets Equal (aspartame) sugar substitute

Stir together cocoa, cornstarch, dry milk, and salt to blend in a small saucepan. Stir water into dry mixture until smooth. Add margarine and cook and stir over low heat. Bring to a boil and simmer for 2 minutes, stirring constantly. Remove from heat.

Add vanilla and sweetener to sauce. Stir lightly to mix. Pour into a glass jar and refrigerate until used. Return to room temperature before serving over ice cream, or it may be heated again to serve on cake or pudding. Serve 2 tablespoons per serving.

Nutritive values per serving:	CAL	CHO (gm)	PRO (gm)	FAT (gm)	NA (mg)
	31	3	1	2	52

Food exchanges per serving: ½ vegetable
Low-sodium diets: Omit salt.

16
COOKIES

A friend of mine commented when I started this book that she would like me to include some crisp cookies. She said that she was so tired of the soft cookies, which were all she knew how to make. I've never been too fond of those, either, so I tried to work on some rather crisp cookies. Sugar helps, but since we can't have much of that we need something else to give us that crisp texture. Egg whites also help, so I used those in several recipes; and believe it or not, just letting the cookies sit on a tray at room temperature for a couple of days helps. The buttermilk cookies in this chapter, which I'm very proud of, become much more crisp after you let them stay out for a couple of days.

I like to have cookies on hand for special occasions and therefore I generally try to keep some cookies in the freezer. All of the cookies in this chapter freeze well because I don't consider a cookie that can't be frozen very practical. If I'm having company and they don't need diabetic cookies, I always include some of my own cookies on the tray so I can have a cookie or two without comment—although it is amazing how many people tell me they would like to cut down on sugar and choose to eat my cookies instead of the ones with lots of sugar and fat in them.

Since our cookies need to be low cholesterol as well as low carbohydrate, we need to make them without butter, cream, whole milk, egg yolks, lard, chocolate, and coconut. I'm glad we can have cocoa, nuts, raisins, applesauce, and other fruits, even if we do have to count them, because we can use all of those to make our cookies more interesting. Cookies can't be frosted with powdered sugar frosting or rolled in powdered sugar, but they can be rolled in granular sugar substitute, which works rather well.

Of course, while we are making our diabetic low-cholesterol cookies, we still need to observe the fundamentals of good cookie-making. I have found that following these guidelines helps me to have better cookies:

1. Read the recipe to be sure you understand it before you start. Get out all of the ingredients and any equipment you will need to make the cookies before you start mixing any ingredients. I generally start preheating the oven after I am sure I have everything ready to go, since I need to preheat my oven for 10 minutes and that is about the length of time it takes me to mix up a batch of cookies.

2. Use good quality ingredients and don't substitute ingredients without regard to the proper substitution rates.

3. Don't sift flour unless the recipe tells you to do so because sifted and unsifted flours measure differently. I almost never sift flour. Flour is sifted to mix it with other ingredients and to make it lighter, and both of these are accomplished when it is stirred.

4. Always use regulation measuring cups and spoons. Cakes and cookies are delicately balanced formulas and won't respond well to irregular measurements.

5. It is important that ingredients should be at room temperature if the recipe so indicates. This is especially important for liquid egg substitute and margarine.

6. All cookies on the same baking sheet should be the same size and thickness so they will bake evenly. If there is not enough dough for a full pan of cookies, bake them on a smaller pan or in the center of the larger pan you have been using.

7. Cookies should be placed on a cool pan before they are put in the oven. A hot pan will start them baking before they go in the oven and will generally result in imperfectly baked cookies. Cookies should also be loosened from hot pans and put on a wire rack to cool so they won't continue baking after they are removed from the oven.

8. Cookies should be defrosted in the container in which they were frozen or in another airtight container so they don't pick up moisture from the air, which softens them. If they are to be defrosted on a plate, the plate should be refrigerated so they can defrost at the temperature in the refrigerator and not at room temperature.

BROWNIES

Yields 2 dozen squares—24 servings

I'm a chocoholic so you know I tried very hard to develop a recipe for brownies that I could eat. We like these best made with the black walnuts that grow so abundantly in this area, but they are also good with pecans or other types of nuts.

½ **cup cocoa**
⅓ **cup boiling water**
2 cups all-purpose flour
1 teaspoon baking soda
½ **teaspoon salt**
4 large egg whites at room temperature
2 teaspoons vanilla
Liquid sugar substitute equal to ½ cup sugar
½ **cup white corn syrup**
1 cup (2 sticks) margarine at room temperature
1 cup chopped nuts

Mix together cocoa and boiling water with a teaspoon until smooth and set aside to cool to room temperature. Place flour, soda, and salt in mixer bowl and mix at low speed about 1 minute to blend well. Add egg whites, vanilla, sugar substitute, and corn syrup to cocoa mixture and mix with a spoon to blend. Add margarine to flour mixture along with cocoa mixture and mix at medium speed about 1 minute or until well blended. Do not overmix.

Add nuts to dough. Spread dough evenly (this is very important) in a 11″ × 15″ jelly roll pan that has been greased with margarine or sprayed with pan spray. Bake at 350° F. for about 20 minutes, or until the brownies start to pull away from the sides of the pan. Cool to room temperature and cut 4 × 6 to yield 24 squares. Serve 1 square per serving.

Nutritive values per serving:	CAL	CHO (gm)	PRO (gm)	FAT (gm)	NA (mg)
	167	15	3	11	199

Food exchanges per serving: 1 bread, 2 fat
Low-sodium diets: Omit salt. Use salt-free margarine and unsalted nuts.

CHOCOLATE BALLS

Yields 20 cookies—10 servings

This cookie, based on a recipe from Frances Nielsen, is one of my sister Shirley's favorites. I hesitated to include it because it didn't seem to me that I got that much for my bread exchange, but she liked it so well that I decided to use it.

½ **cup (1 stick) margarine at room temperature**
2 **tablespoons sugar**
2 **teaspoons vanilla**
Liquid sugar substitute equal to ⅓ **cup sugar**
1¼ **cups all-purpose flour**
3 **tablespoons cocoa**
½ **teaspoon salt**
¼ **cup chopped nuts**
2 **tablespoons raisins**
Sprinkle Sweet granulated sugar substitute as necessary

Cream together margarine and sugar until light and fluffy. Add vanilla and sugar substitute to creamed mixture. Beat at medium speed for ½ minute. Stir together flour, cocoa, and salt to blend. Add to creamed mixture and mix at low speed about 1 minute or until blended.

Add nuts and raisins to dough. Mix lightly. Shape into balls using 1 tablespoonful of dough per ball. Place balls on a cookie sheet that has been lined with aluminum foil or sprayed with pan spray. Bake at 325° F. for 20–25 minutes or until slightly firm. Remove from oven and cool slightly.

Roll lukewarm balls in Sprinkle Sweet. Cool to room temperature, and serve 2 balls per serving.

VARIATION: CHOCOLATE MINT BALLS
Add ½ teaspoon peppermint flavoring along with 1 teaspoon vanilla instead of the 2 teaspoons vanilla.

Nutritive values per serving:	CAL	CHO (gm)	PRO (gm)	FAT (gm)	NA (mg)
	178	16	2	11	155

Food exchanges per serving: 1 bread, 2 fat
Low-sodium diets: Omit salt. Use salt-free margarine and unsalted nuts.

CHOCOLATE CHIP COOKIES

Yields 3 dozen cookies—18 servings

1 cup (2 sticks) margarine at room temperature
¼ cup sugar
¾ cup Brown Sugar Twin sugar substitute
3 large egg whites at room temperature
1 tablespoon vanilla
2 cups all-purpose flour
1 teaspoon baking soda
¼ teaspoon salt
¼ cup water at room temperature
½ cup mini semisweet chocolate chips

Cream margarine, sugar, and sugar substitute at medium speed until light and fluffy. Add egg whites and vanilla to creamed mixture and beat at medium speed for 1 minute.

Stir together flour, soda, and salt to blend well. Add ¼ cup water to creamed mixture along with the flour mixture and mix at medium speed for 1 minute or until smooth.

Add chocolate chips to dough and mix lightly. Drop by tablespoonful onto cookie sheets that have been lined with aluminum foil or sprayed with pan spray. Press down lightly with fingers dipped in cold water to form a circle about 2 inches across. Bake at 375° F. for about 12 minutes or until browned. (The cookies won't be crisp unless they are browned.) Remove cookies from hot cookie sheets to wire racks to cool to room temperature. Allow 2 cookies per serving.

VARIATION: CHOCOLATE CHIP BARS
Instead of dropping dough onto cookie sheets, spread dough evenly in a jelly roll pan (11" × 15") that has been greased with margarine or sprayed with pan spray. Bake at 375° F. for 20 to 25 minutes, or until lightly browned and the bars pull away from the sides of the pan. Cool to room temperature and cut 9 × 4 to yield 36 bars. Serve 2 bars per serving.

Nutritive values per serving:	CAL	CHO (gm)	PRO (gm)	FAT (gm)	NA (mg)
	180	18	3	12	220

Food exchanges per serving: 1 bread, 2 fat (Exchanges remain the same for the variation of the basic recipe)

Low-sodium diets: Omit salt. Use salt-free margarine.

MOCHA COOKIES

Yields 18 cookies—18 servings

These cookies are a favorite of our neighbor, Jan Franks, who likes cookies very much and especially these. We have them often with a cup of coffee and a good visit.

½ cup (1 stick) margarine at room temperature
2 tablespoons sugar
2 teaspoons vanilla
Liquid sugar substitute equal to ⅓ cup sugar
1¼ cups all-purpose flour
3 tablespoons cocoa
2 teaspoons dry instant or freeze-dried coffee
1 teaspoon baking powder
¼ cup raisins
¼ cup chopped nuts
2 large egg whites at room temperature

Cream together margarine and sugar until light and fluffy. Add vanilla and sugar substitute to creamed mixture and mix lightly. Stir together flour, cocoa, coffee, and baking powder to blend. Add to creamed mixture and mix at medium speed 1–2 minutes or until blended. Add raisins and nuts to dough and mix lightly.

Add egg whites to dough and mix until egg whites are absorbed into the dough. Drop dough by the tablespoonful onto a cookie sheet that has been lined with aluminum foil or sprayed with pan spray. Using your fingers dipped in cold water, shape the dough into round cookies about ¼ inch thick. Spread the dough carefully because the finished cookie will be the shape of the dough after it is baked. Bake at 375° F. about 12 minutes or until the dough springs back when touched. Transfer from the hot cookie sheet onto a wire rack and cool to room temperature. Serve 1 cookie per serving.

Nutritive values per serving:	CAL	CHO (gm)	PRO (gm)	FAT (gm)	NA (mg)
	104	10	2	6	95

Food exchanges per serving: ½ bread, 1 fat
Low-sodium diets: Use salt-free margarine, low-sodium baking
    powder, and unsalted nuts.

BUTTERMILK COOKIES

Yields 30 cookies—15 servings

These cookies are based on a recipe for buttermilk cookies that Vera Wilson has been making for years. I have always loved them and she used to save some of them for me whenever she or her daughter Mary made them. I hated to give them up when I became diabetic, but I feel better about it now that I have developed a cookie suitable for my diet that is almost like the original.

½ cup (1 stick) margarine at room temperature
¼ cup sugar
2 teaspoons vanilla
Liquid sugar substitute equal to ⅓ cup sugar
½ cup liquid egg substitute at room temperature
2 cups all-purpose flour
½ teaspoon baking soda
½ teaspoon baking powder
2 tablespoons dry buttermilk
1 to 2 tablespoons water

Cream together margarine and sugar until light and fluffy. Add vanilla, sugar substitute, and egg substitute to creamed mixture and beat at medium speed for 1 minute. Stir together flour, soda, baking powder, and dry buttermilk to blend and add to creamed mixture.

Add to creamed and flour mixture as much of the water as necessary to make a soft dough. While adding, beat at low speed. Roll out on a lightly floured working surface to about ¼-inch thickness. Cut with a 3-inch cookie cutter and place on cookie sheets that have been lined with aluminum foil or sprayed with pan spray. Sprinkle with Cinnamon Shake (see index) if desired and bake at 350° F. for 12–15 minutes or until lightly browned. (The cookies need to be browned on the bottom to develop their best flavor.) Remove from hot cookie sheets to wire rack and cool to room temperature. Serve 2 cookies to a serving.

VARIATIONS:
SPICE COOKIES: Add 1 teaspoon pumpkin pie spice, apple pie spice, or cinnamon along with the flour.
CHOCOLATE COOKIES: Use ¼ cup cocoa and 1¾ cups all-purpose flour instead of the 2 cups all-purpose flour in the basic recipe.
PASTEL COOKIES: Substitute ¼ cup fruit-flavored regular, non-diabetic gelatin for the ¼ cup sugar in the basic recipe.

Nutritive values per serving:	CAL	CHO (gm)	PRO (gm)	FAT (gm)	NA (mg)
	140	16	2	7	134

Food exchanges per serving: 1 bread, 1 fat (Exchanges remain the same for variations of the basic recipe)

Low-sodium diets: Use salt-free margarine and low-sodium baking powder.

OATMEAL COOKIES

Yields 3 dozen cookies—36 servings

Vera Wilson says that this cookie (with lots more sugar in it, of course) is one that she has been making ever since her oldest daughter Donna was just a baby. I like it especially well because it reminds me of the oatmeal cookies that my mother used to make when we were children. She also used to send them to me at college, and later to my sister and me when we were living in Chicago.

⅓ **cup raisins**
¾ **cup boiling water**
2 **tablespoons sugar**
2 **teaspoons Weight Watcher's granulated sugar substitute**
1 **cup (2 sticks) margarine at room temperature**
½ **cup liquid egg substitute at room temperature**
1 **teaspoon vanilla**
2 **cups all-purpose flour**
1 **teaspoon cinnamon**
1 **teaspoon baking powder**
½ **teaspoon baking soda**
2 **cups rolled oats or rolled wheat**
½ **cup chopped nuts**

Combine raisins and boiling water and set aside to cool to room temperature.

Cream together sugar, sugar substitute, and margarine at medium speed until light and fluffy. Add egg substitute and vanilla to creamed mixture and mix at low speed for 1 minute.

Stir together flour, cinnamon, baking powder, and soda to blend well.

Add oats and nuts to creamed mixture along with flour mixture, raisins, and liquid in which raisins were soaked. Mix at medium speed until flour is moistened. Drop by heaping tablespoonful onto cookie sheets that have been lined with aluminum foil or sprayed with pan spray. Press down lightly with fingers dipped in cold water to form circles about 2 inches across; bake at 375° F. for 10–12 minutes. Remove from hot cookie sheet to wire rack to cool to room temperature. Serve 1 cookie per serving.

Nutritive values per serving:

	CAL	CHO (gm)	PRO (gm)	FAT (gm)	NA (mg)
	107	11	2	7	94

Food exchanges per serving: 1 bread, 1 fat

Low-sodium diets: Use salt-free margarine, low-sodium baking powder, and unsalted nuts.

DATE GRAHAM COOKIES

Yields 2 dozen cookies—24 servings

These cookies have fiber in the graham flour and also in the dates.

1 cup graham flour
½ cup all-purpose flour
3 tablespoons dry buttermilk
½ teaspoon baking soda
½ teaspoon salt
½ cup Brown Sugar Twin sugar substitute
2 large egg whites at room temperature
¼ cup dark molasses
½ cup (1 stick) margarine at room temperature
½ cup chopped dates

Place flours, dry buttermilk, soda, salt, and sugar substitute in mixer bowl and mix at low speed for about 1 minute to mix well. Add egg whites, molasses, and margarine to flour mixture and mix at medium speed for about 1 minute or until well blended.

Add dates to dough and mix lightly. Drop by tablespoonful onto cookie sheets that have been lined with aluminum foil or sprayed with pan spray. Bake at 375° F. for 10–12 minutes, or until lightly browned. Remove from hot cookie sheets onto wire rack to cool to room temperature. Serve 1 cookie per serving.

Nutritive values per serving:

	CAL	CHO (gm)	PRO (gm)	FAT (gm)	NA (mg)
	83	11	2	4	125

Food exchanges per serving: 1 bread, 1 fat

Low-sodium diets: Omit salt. Use salt-free margarine.

WHOLE WHEAT SPICE COOKIES

Yields 2 dozen cookies—24 servings

½ cup (1 stick) margarine at room temperature
¼ cup brown sugar
2 teaspoons vanilla
Liquid sugar substitute equal to ⅓ cup sugar
3 large egg whites at room temperature
2 tablespoons water at room temperature
⅔ cup whole wheat flour
1⅓ cups all-purpose flour
½ teaspoon baking soda
½ teaspoon baking powder
¼ teaspoon salt
1 teaspoon cinnamon
½ teaspoon nutmeg
2 tablespoons dry buttermilk

Cream together margarine and sugar until light and fluffy. Add vanilla, sugar substitute, egg whites, and water to creamed mixture and mix 2 minutes at medium speed.

Stir together remaining dry ingredients to blend well. Add to creamed mixture and mix at low speed to blend. Roll on a lightly floured working surface to ¼-inch thickness. Cut with a 3-inch cookie cutter and place on cookie sheets that have been lined with aluminum foil or sprayed with pan spray. Bake at 350° F. for 12–15 minutes, or until lightly browned. Remove from hot cookie sheet to wire rack and cool to room temperature. Serve 1 cookie per serving.

Nutritive values per serving:

	CAL	CHO (gm)	PRO (gm)	FAT (gm)	NA (mg)
	85	10	2	4	107

Food exchanges per serving: ½ bread, 1 fat
Low-sodium diets: Omit salt. Use salt-free margarine and low-sodium baking powder.

PEANUT BUTTER COOKIES

Yields 30 cookies—15 servings

This recipe from Frances Nielsen can be made with smooth peanut butter, but we prefer chunky.

½ **cup chunky peanut butter at room temperature**
⅓ **cup (⅔ stick) margarine at room temperature**
¼ **cup dark molasses**
2 teaspoons liquid sugar substitute
3 large egg whites at room temperature
1¼ **cups all-purpose flour**
½ **teaspoon baking soda**
⅛ **teaspoon salt**

Cream together peanut butter, margarine, molasses, and sugar substitute at medium speed until smooth. Add egg whites to creamed mixture and beat at medium speed until smooth.

Stir together flour, soda, and salt to blend and add to creamed mixture. Mix at medium speed until smooth. Drop by tablespoonful onto a cookie sheet that has been lined with aluminum foil or sprayed with pan spray. Press down lightly with fingers dipped in cold water to form circles about 2 inches wide. Bake at 375° F. for 10–12 minutes, or until lightly browned. Remove from hot cookie sheet to wire rack and cool to room temperature. Serve 2 cookies per serving.

Nutritive values per serving:	CAL	CHO (gm)	PRO (gm)	FAT (gm)	NA (mg)
	140	13	4	9	169

Food exchanges per serving: 1 bread, 2 fat
Low-sodium diets: Omit salt. Use salt-free peanut butter and margarine.

HIGH-FIBER COOKIES

Yields 4 dozen cookies—48 servings

These cookies, which provide 2 grams of dietary fiber each, aren't terribly sweet. We like them this way, but if you prefer them sweeter, you can add 1 tablespoon of Weight Watchers dry substitute when you add the sugar without changing the nutritive values.

1 cup oat bran
1 cup rolled oats
1 cup Fiber One cereal
1 cup Kellogg's Bran Flakes
1 cup seedless raisins
1 cup chopped English walnuts
¾ cup sugar
¾ cup brown sugar
1 cup (2 sticks) margarine
2 large egg whites
2 teaspoons vanilla
2 cups all-purpose flour
1 teaspoon baking powder
1 teaspoon soda
½ teaspoon salt
½ cup water at room temperature

Place oat bran, rolled oats, Fiber One, Bran Flakes, raisins, and walnuts in a bowl. Mix lightly and set aside.

Place sugars and margarine in mixer bowl and mix at medium speed until light and fluffy. Add egg whites and vanilla and mix lightly, scraping down bowl before and after adding egg whites and vanilla.

In a separate bowl combine flour, baking powder, soda, and salt and mix at low speed about ½ minute to blend well. Add flour mixture and water to sugar mixture and mix at medium speed only until flour is moistened. Add bran mixture and mix at medium speed until well blended.

Drop by heaping tablespoonfuls onto a cookie sheet that has been sprayed with cooking spray or lined with aluminum foil. Bake at 375° F. for 12–14 minutes or until lightly browned. Remove from oven and let sit for 1 minute. Remove cookies to a wire rack and cool to room temperature. Serve 1 cookie per serving.

Nutritive values per serving:

	CAL	CHO (gm)	PRO (gm)	FAT (gm)	NA (mg)
	121	15	2	6	107

Food exchanges per serving: 1 bread, 1 fat
Low-sodium diets: May be used as written.

MEXICAN WEDDING COOKIES

Yields 3 dozen cookies—36 servings

These cookies are based on a recipe from Frances Nielsen. They freeze beautifully and look so nice when they are rolled in the Sprinkle Sweet.

1½ cups (3 sticks) margarine at room temperature
½ cup powdered sugar
2 teaspoons vanilla
Liquid sugar substitute equal to ⅓ cup sugar
3 cups all-purpose flour
¾ cup chopped nuts
Sprinkle Sweet granulated sugar substitute as necessary

Cream together margarine and powdered sugar at medium speed until light and fluffy. Add vanilla, sugar substitute, and flour to creamed mixture and mix at medium speed about 2 minutes or until well blended.

Add nuts to dough and mix at low speed only until nuts are blended into the dough. Form dough into balls using a heaping tablespoon of dough for each ball. Bake on cookie sheets lined with aluminum foil or sprayed with pan spray at 350° F. for about 20 minutes, or until lightly browned. Remove from heat.

Roll cookies in Sprinkle Sweet while they are warm but not hot.

Nutritive values per serving:

	CAL	CHO (gm)	PRO (gm)	FAT (gm)	NA (mg)
	129	10	2	9	96

Food exchanges per serving: ½ bread, 2 fat
Low-sodium diets: Use salt-free margarine and unsalted nuts.

NUT SLICES

Yields 2 dozen cookies—24 servings

This recipe is based on one from Anita Kane of Shorewood, Wisconsin. We trade recipes frequently and hers are always so good. I would always feel safe giving away a copy of one of her recipes without testing it, because I know that she has tested it thoroughly before giving it to me.

½ **cup (1 stick) margarine at room temperature**
2 **tablespoons sugar**
4 **large egg whites at room temperature**
Liquid sugar substitute equal to ⅓ **cup sugar**
1 **teaspoon vanilla**
½ **teaspoon almond flavoring**
2 **cups all-purpose flour**
1 **teaspoon baking powder**
½ **teaspoon salt**
½ **cup chopped almonds**

Cream together margarine and sugar until light and fluffy. Add egg whites, sugar substitute, vanilla, and almond flavoring to creamed mixture and mix at medium speed about 1 minute to blend. Add flour, baking powder, and salt to creamed mixture and mix at medium speed for 1 minute or until well blended.

Add almonds to dough. Turn out onto a lightly floured working surface and form into a roll about 2 inches wide and 12 inches long. Flatten the top of the roll, keeping it the same size, and place on a cookie sheet that has been lined with aluminum foil or sprayed with pan spray. Bake at 350° F. for 25 minutes. Remove roll from hot cookie sheet onto a working surface. As soon as you can handle the roll, slice with a serrated knife into 24 slices about ½ inch thick. Place the slices flat on the cookie sheet and return to the 350° F. oven. Bake 5 minutes on one side and then about the same on the other side. Remove from hot cookie sheet to a cooling rack and cool to room temperature. Serve 1 slice per serving.

Note: If another kind of nut is used other than almonds, use another flavoring instead of the almond flavoring. We use black walnuts in this area and I'm sure that everyone has their own favorites.

Nutritive values per serving:	CAL	CHO (gm)	PRO (gm)	FAT (gm)	NA (mg)
	95	10	2	5	110

Food exchanges per serving: ½ bread, 1 fat
Low-sodium diets: Omit salt. Use salt-free margarine, low-sodium baking powder, and unsalted nuts.

RAISIN BARS

Yields 20 squares—20 servings

This recipe is based on one from Vera Wilson. Her recipe is richer and is frosted, but I'm sure you will like this version, also.

⅓ **cup raisins**
1 cup water
¾ **cup (1½ sticks) margarine at room temperature**
¼ **cup sugar**
3 large egg whites at room temperature
Liquid sugar substitute equal to ½ cup sugar
2¼ **cups all-purpose flour**
1 teaspoon baking soda
½ **teaspoon salt**
1 teaspoon cinnamon

Combine raisins and water in a small saucepan. Bring to a boil, cover, and remove from heat. Cool to room temperature.

Cream together margarine and sugar until light and fluffy. Add egg whites and sugar substitute to creamed mixture and mix at medium speed for 1 minute.

Stir together flour, soda, salt, and cinnamon to blend well. Add to creamed mixture along with the raisins and the liquid in which they were cooked. Mix at medium speed about 1 minute or until well blended. Spread evenly in a 9″ × 13″ cake pan that has been well greased with margarine. Bake at 350° F. for 25–30 minutes or until browned and the bars pull away from the sides of the pan. Cut 4 × 5 to yield 20 squares. Serve 1 square per serving.

Nutritive values per serving:	CAL	CHO (gm)	PRO (gm)	FAT (gm)	NA (mg)
	132	16	2	7	197

Food exchanges per serving: 1 bread, 1 fat
Low-sodium diets: Omit salt and use salt-free margarine.

APPLESAUCE BRAN SQUARES

Yields 15 squares—15 servings

This recipe is based on one from Betty Jane Walter of Jackson, Michigan. Betty Jane is a dietary consultant as well as a diabetic and we often discuss our work as well as our favorite recipes. She has been very active in the American Heart Association program in her area and is concerned about low-cholesterol diets as well as diabetic diets.

1 cup all-purpose flour
²/₃ cup Bran Buds, All Bran, or 100% Bran
½ cup rolled oats
2 tablespoons brown sugar
½ teaspoon salt
½ teaspoon baking soda
1 teaspoon baking powder
1 teaspoon cinnamon
¼ teaspoon cloves or nutmeg
½ cup (1 stick) margarine at room temperature
2 large egg whites at room temperature
1 teaspoon vanilla
Liquid sugar substitute equal to ½ cup sugar
¹/₃ cup chopped nuts
1 cup unsweetened applesauce at room temperature

Place dry ingredients in mixer bowl and mix at low speed for 1 minute.

Add margarine, egg whites, vanilla, sugar substitute, nuts, and applesauce to flour mixture and mix at medium speed for ½ minute or until blended. Spread evenly in a 9″ × 13″ cake pan which has been greased with margarine or sprayed with pan spray. Bake at 375° F. for 25–30 minutes or until browned and it starts to pull away from the sides of the pan. Cut 3 × 5 into 15 squares and serve warm or at room temperature. Serve 1 square per serving.

Nutritive values per serving:	CAL	CHO (gm)	PRO (gm)	FAT (gm)	NA (mg)
	135	14	3	8	240

Food exchanges per serving: 1 bread, 1½ fat
Low-sodium diets: Omit salt. Use salt-free margarine, low-sodium baking powder, and salt-free nuts.

17
BEVERAGES

A good hot beverage or a well-chilled sugar-free soft drink can be a real lift when you are hot and tired—or cold and tired, too, for that matter. Beverages are such a part of our lives that we need to know what we can enjoy without going off our diet when we want something to drink. I used to hate those sugar-free soft drinks that were available, but now that they are sweetened with NutraSweet I find that I really enjoy them.

It is also nice to have beverages you can serve for parties or when friends drop in. I make my own low-calorie cocoa mix that I think is extra special. A friend of mine who was counting her calories asked for some of it the other day, and she told me she liked it even better than the regular commercial kind I had given our husbands. She took my recipe home with her and said she was going to make it up for herself to enjoy when she needed a pickup or had guests.

When you go to a party and it seems like food and socializing always go together, you can always walk around with a cup of black coffee or a glass of iced tea or sugar-free soft drink and have just as much fun as anyone else.

If you are home alone and hungry or thirsty and don't want to spend any more of your exchanges, you can have a twist of lemon in ice water (which is one of my favorites), or a cup of hot bouillon or tomato juice with a twist of lemon in it. Last fall when I was visiting Bud and Frances Gunsallus in Miami, I discovered that half of a lime from the tree in their backyard put a lot of life into a glass of ice water or sugar-free 7-Up.

In other words, use what is available in the line of sugarless beverages and have just as much fun as everyone else at the party—or get a real lift when you are tired and just need a pickup.

SPARKLING PUNCH

Yields 1 gallon—32 4-ounce cups

The first time I talked to Mary Agnes Jones and the other dietitians at Holy Cross Hospital in Chicago about this book, they told me that one thing that was high on the list of recipes they needed was a punch that would be free for diabetics. I think this answers that need very well. It's not only free, it's also delicious.

2 .14- or .20-ounce packets of Wyler's unsweetened flavored soft drink mix or Kool-Aid unsweetened soft drink mix (2-quart size)
1 quart water
3 quarts chilled sugar-free 7-Up or sugar-free ginger ale

Dissolve drink mix in water and refrigerate until needed. Place in punch bowl along with a chunk of ice.

Add 7-Up or ginger ale to drink mix in bowl. Mix lightly and serve a 4-ounce cup per serving.

I like to freeze some of the drink mix (which has been prepared with water according to directions on the package) in a bowl or plastic container to be used instead of ice in the punch bowl. This keeps the punch from being diluted as the ice melts. To add a special touch, you can add a few grapes or strawberries in with the mix you are freezing.

Nutritive values per serving:	Negligible
Food exchanges per serving:	None (It may be used as desired without counting any exchanges)
Low-sodium diets:	May be used as written

HOT SPICED TEA

Yields 15 cups—30 servings

This recipe is from Edith Robinson, a dietitian from Decatur, Georgia. Edith and I worked together at the Army Food Service Center in Chicago. She told me that she got the recipe from our commanding officer Colonel Cozad's wife, who served it one cold day when she and Colonel Cozad entertained the members of the department at their home.

12 cups water
1 teaspoon whole cloves
4 sticks cinnamon
6 tea bags
¼ cup lemon juice
1 cup unsweetened pineapple juice
1½ cups unsweetened orange juice
Sugar substitute equal to ¾ cup sugar

Combine water, cloves, and cinnamon and simmer, covered, for 5 minutes. Remove from heat. Add tea bags to hot liquid and steep for 5 minutes. Remove tea bags and spices.

Add juices to tea and mix lightly. Tea may be cooled to room temperature and refrigerated overnight at this stage, if desired. If tea is refrigerated, it should be reheated before it is served.

Add sugar substitute just before tea is served. Taste for flavor and add a little more lemon juice or sugar substitute, if desired. Serve 1 4-ounce punch cup per serving.

	CAL	CHO (gm)	PRO (gm)	FAT (gm)	NA (mg)
Nutritive values per serving:	11	3	negl.	negl.	negl.

Food exchanges per serving: 2 servings is 1 vegetable exchange (1 serving may be considered free)

Low-sodium diets: May be used as written

HOT COCOA MIX

Yields mix for 32 6-ounce cups of cocoa

¾ cup cocoa
½ teaspoon salt
1 quart instant dry milk
Dry sugar substitute equal to 1–1½ cups sugar

Mix ingredients well and store in an airtight container in a moderately cool place. Use 2 tablespoons mix plus 6 ounces boiling water for 1 6-ounce serving of cocoa.

VARIATIONS:
MEXICAN COCOA: Add 2–3 teaspoons ground cinnamon when mixing the total ingredients; or place a scant ⅛ teaspoon of cinnamon in a cup, 2 tablespoons of the mix, and 6 ounces boiling water for 1 serving.
MOCHA: Add ⅓ cup instant coffee when mixing the total ingredients; or place ½ teaspoon instant coffee in a cup, 2 tablespoons of the mix, and 6 ounces boiling water for 1 serving.

Nutritive values per serving:	CAL	CHO (gm)	PRO (gm)	FAT (gm)	NA (mg)
	49	4	3	3	113

Food exchanges per serving:　⅓ milk, ½ fat
Low-sodium diets:　Omit salt.

CHOCOLATE MILK SHAKE

Yields 1 milk shake

This recipe from Patti Dillon, our Fayette County home economics extension agent, is cool and refreshing and costs a lot less in calories and exchanges than you would expect.

1 cup skim milk
2 teaspoons cocoa
1 1-gram packet Equal (aspartame) sugar substitute
3 or 4 ice cubes

Place ingredients in blender or food processor and beat at high speed until frothy and thickened. Serve immediately. Total amount is 1 serving.

Nutritive values per serving:	CAL	CHO (gm)	PRO (gm)	FAT (gm)	NA (mg)
	97	14	9	negl.	154
Food exchanges per serving:	1 milk				
Low-sodium diets:	Use as written.				

CHOCOLATE LIQUEUR

Yields 1 quart—32 1-ounce servings

I like to sprinkle a couple of tablespoons of this over a chocolate cake before I cut it and put the topping on it. It adds a certain something to the cake without increasing the food value very much. In fact, 3 tablespoons on one cake doesn't need to be counted since the amount per portion is so small. Gail Olson of Volga City, Iowa, gave me this recipe and the one following. They are both good over ice milk or served with an after-dinner drink.

2 cups vodka
1½ cups water
1½ cups Brown Sugar Twin sugar substitute
4 ounces chocolate extract
2 teaspoons vanilla
½ teaspoon peppermint extract (optional)

Combine ingredients and pour into a dark-colored glass bottle. Let set for 2 weeks before it is used. Store as you would any liqueur. Consider 1 ounce (2 tablespoons) per serving when calculating nutritional values.

Nutritive values per serving:	CAL	CHO (gm)	PRO (gm)	FAT (gm)	NA (mg)
	37	negl.	negl.	negl.	negl.
Food exchanges per serving:	1 fat				
Low-sodium diets:	May be used as written.				

ORANGE LIQUEUR

Yields 1 quart—32 1-ounce servings

Frances Nielsen had taught me to appreciate the flavor of fruit and orange liqueur combined together, using about 1 tablespoon orange liqueur per serving of fruit. I had given that up because of the high carbohydrate content of liqueurs until Gail Olson of Volga City, Iowa, gave me this recipe. It is good over ice milk or served as an after-dinner drink and is also marvelous with fruit.

2 cups water
Thin peel from 2 large oranges
2 teaspoons vanilla
1 teaspoon lemon flavoring
2 teaspoons orange flavoring
1 drop yellow food color
1 drop orange food color
2 cups vodka
Sugar substitute equal to ½ cup sugar

Combine water and orange peel and simmer, covered, over low heat for 5 minutes. Cool to room temperature.

Add remaining ingredients to simmered mixture. Pour into a glass or stainless steel container. Cover and keep in a dark place for 2 weeks. Strain and discard any solids. Pour into a dark glass bottle and store as you would any liqueur. Consider 1 ounce (2 tablespoons) per serving when calculating nutritional values.

Nutritive values per serving:	CAL	CHO (gm)	PRO (gm)	FAT (gm)	NA (mg)
	37	negl.	negl.	negl.	negl.
Food exchanges per serving:	1 fat				
Low-sodium diets:	May be used as written				

18
CANNING AND FREEZING FOODS

If you have been canning and freezing fruits and vegetables, don't stop now. This is a good time to take advantage of your expertise to save yourself some money. Canning for the low-cholesterol diabetic diet is no more complicated than any other kind of canning. The canned fruits and vegetables you buy in the store canned without sugar or salt are just that—the same items you have always canned—only this time you don't want to add any sugar (or any salt if you are on a low-sodium diet) to the canned foods. Neither sugar nor salt is necessary for preservation of canned or frozen foods and it is simple to can without them.

Sugar helps fruit develop the characteristic color, flavor, aroma, and shape which we associate with canned fruit. Fruit canned without sugar will be softer—which isn't all that bad—and may have a little more delicate coloring, but it is an excellent product and one that you will enjoy using long after you can it. I have always enjoyed seeing jars of fruits, vegetables, and pickles on my shelves, and there is no reason why I can't go on doing it—even if they can't have much sugar in them.

When we are canning for the low-cholesterol diabetic diet, we need only worry about the diabetic part of the diet. The only canned item I can think of that includes any cholesterol is mincemeat, which is made with suet. You can handle that by canning mincemeat without sugar or suet and adding some margarine and sugar substitute when you are ready to use it.

Use ripe, firm fruit for the best flavor. It can be canned in fruit juice or in plain water. If you want to can fruit in its own juice, thoroughly crush the fruit, cover it with water, and bring it to a boil over low heat. Strain it through a clean cloth and use the juice for canning.

Fruit may also be packed with unsweetened juice of another kind—for instance, pears canned in unsweetened pineapple juice or peaches canned in unsweetened orange juice. The fruit juice needs to be counted as a separate exchange when you drink it or use it with the fruit, if it is consumed in an amount equal to a fruit exchange. For water-packed fruit, ½ cup is 1 fruit exchange. However, for juice-packed fruit, ⅓ cup drained fruit is equal to 1 fruit exchange and the juice would be calculated according to the type of juice you used.

When I want a more flavorful water-packed fruit, I open the jar a couple of days before I want to use it. I add ½ teaspoon lemon juice per cup of fruit and sugar substitute to taste to sweeten the juice. Then I return it to the refrigerator until I need it. It really improves the flavor of the fruit. This does not change the fruit exchanges—it is still ½ cup of fruit per fruit exchange—but it adds a lot to the flavor of the fruit.

Half-pint or pint jars are usually the best to use for water-packed fruit, unless several persons will be eating it. Half-pint jars should be processed the same length of time as pint jars. I also like to use the 1½-cup jars, which are also processed the same length of time as pint jars. Some 3-cup jars are also available now, which require the same processing time as quart jars.

Procedures for canning fruit without sugar are the same as for canning fruit with sugar, except that water is added to the jars instead of a sugar syrup. Important points to remember are as follows:

- *Choose ripe but firm fruit.* If you purchase fruit to can, try to get it as soon after it is picked as possible. It is a good idea to buy it from a nearby garden or orchard. Use only perfect fruit. Remember, there is a lot of fiber in the skin of apples and plums and use it if at all possible. Sort fruit for size and ripeness, using like fruits together if you are canning different fruits.
- *Wash all fruit thoroughly* even if it is going to be pared. Dirt contains bacteria. Wash fruits a small amount at a time, taking the fruit out of the water instead of pouring the water off the fruit. Use several changes of water and rinse the pan thoroughly between washings. Do not let fruits soak because they will lose their flavor and some food value, and handle them gently to prevent bruising.

- *To prevent darkening* use an ascorbic acid mix (available in grocery and drug stores) according to instructions on the container, or drop the peeled fruit into water containing 2 teaspoons each of salt and vinegar per gallon of water. Drain this liquid off the fruit before the fruit is canned.
- *Hot packing* of fruit is generally preferred. To hot pack fruit, preheat fruit over low heat in a small amount of water or juice, pack into hot jars, and cover with hot liquid. Wipe the rims of the jars, adjust the lids according to manufacturer's directions, and cook in a hot water bath according to directions for the various fruits.
- *Cold pack* is also approved and may be used as desired. If food is to be cold packed, pack the raw fruit in jars, add fruit juice or water, adjust the lid, and cook in a hot water bath according to directions for the various fruits.
- *Processing time* depends upon the fruit to be canned and the size of the containers. The filled jars should be placed in a container with a rack on the bottom under the jars. Add hot water to at least an inch above the top of the jars. The temperature of the water to be added depends upon the temperature of the fruit inside the can. If the fruit was hot packed, the water should be almost boiling hot when it is added. If the fruit was cold packed, the water should be only luke-warm.
- *Head space* should be left between the top of the fruit in the jar and the cover. A knife should be slid between the fruit and the side of the jar before it is sealed to eliminate any air bubbles.
- *Timing* is very important. Start counting processing time when the water in the canner comes to a full rolling boil. Boil gently but steadily for the required time. Add more boiling water if it cooks away during the processing time.
- *Remove jars* from the canner when the canning time is completed. Place the hot jars on a rack or on folded towels. Never place the hot jars on a cold surface because the jars may crack when they touch the cold surface. Keep the hot jars out of drafts and allow them to cool gradually.
- *Check the seals* on the jars the next day. If you have used metal lids, press the top of the lids. If they have sealed they won't move. If they press down when you touch them, the seal is incomplete. After you have checked them, remove the metal rims and wipe the jars clean with a damp cloth, if necessary. If a rim sticks, it will probably help to wrap the lid in a warm, damp cloth for a few moments.
- *If a jar is unsealed or leaking,* use the food soon or can it again. If

you want to can it again, empty the jar and proceed as though it is fresh food you are processing. Before recanning, check the rim of the jar to be sure it is smooth and not cracked, and use a new metal lid.

- *It is a good idea to label each jar* before storing canned goods. I always label jars with the date canned and the contents, and if it is sugar-free I add a note to that effect. For example—*Peaches, July, 1983, W/O sugar*—or without sugar and salt, if that is true.
- *Proper storage* is very important. Jars and other containers should be stored in a cool, dry place. Properly stored foods will keep their quality for a year or more. Canned foods stored near hot pipes, a range, or a furnace, or in direct sunlight may lose eating qualities in a few weeks or months, depending upon the temperature.
- *Be on guard against spoilage.* Do not use canned food with a bulging lid or rim, or a leak. That may mean that the food is spoiled. Also, look for other signs after the jar is opened such as spurting liquid, an off-odor, or mold. When in doubt throw away the food rather than take a chance on it. Spoilage is generally the result of food contamination; being very careful while you are canning will be a big help in preventing spoilage.
- *Jars should be free from nicks and chips.* Home canning jars should be handled carefully. Rough handling can cause tiny cracks and weak spots which could result in jars shattering while the food is being processed. Salad dressing, pickle, and peanut butter jars are not suitable for home canning—they are more likely to break during processing.

The times suggested for keeping the fruit in a hot water bath have changed in recent years and therefore it is wise to check with recent publications for the correct times for each fruit and vegetable. Your library should have some recent information on the subject, and both Kerr and Ball, the makers of glass jars for canning, publish new booklets yearly with all of the latest information in them. These books may be found at libraries, or coupons are available in stores to purchase the current books. The following information was furnished by the Cooperative Extension Service of Iowa State University. If you want more detailed information, you can check with the cooperative extension service in your own state. Remember that timing for water-pack canning is the same for fruit without sugar as for fruit which contains sugar.

I have never been happy with any of the recipes for jams and jellies for diabetics. Many recipes have been published using gelatin as a base but they have to be kept refrigerated and melt as soon as they touch hot toast.

PROCESSING TIMES FOR FRUITS
CANNED IN A WATER BATH

Fruit	Container	Minutes
Apples and applesauce	pints	15
	quarts	20
Apricots, peaches, and pears		
Hot pack	pints	20
	quarts	25
Cold pack	pints	25
	quarts	30
Berries (except strawberries)		
Hot pack for firm berries	pints	10
	quarts	15
Cold pack for soft berries	pints	10
	quarts	15
Cherries		
Hot pack	pints	10
	quarts	15
Cold pack	pints	20
	quarts	25
Fruit juices, except tomato	pints	5
	quarts	5
Plums		
Hot pack	pints	20
	quarts	25
Cold pack	pints	20
	quarts	25
Rhubarb (hot pack)	pints	10
	quarts	10
Tomatoes*		
Hot pack	pints	35
	quarts	45
Cold pack	pints	35
	quarts	45
Tomato juice (hot pack)	pints	35
	quarts	45

The trouble has always been that pectin solidifies only in the presence of sugar, which we can't use. Actually, jellies and jams were the things that I missed the most after I became diabetic. I had always loved jams and jellies and continued to make them after I was married, even though I knew that I could buy ones in the store that were just as good or better than the ones I made.

I am happier now that there are new products on the market which will allow jams and jellies to become firm without sugar. There are several good brands available and I'm sure you can persuade your store to order them, if they aren't carrying them now. Slim Set from MCP Foods is the one that I have been using and I find it very satisfactory, although there are also several other good brands available. Complete directions for making the jams and jellies are included with each page of the jellying agent. An average fruit when made into jam or jelly with Slim Set will give you 8 calories and 2 grams of carbohydrate per tablespoon.

There is very little difference, nutritionally, between vegetables canned at home and vegetables purchased already canned. Several canners are now making low-sodium canned foods available to the public so it is no longer as difficult to follow a low-sodium diet as it used to be. If you want to can low-sodium foods at home, can your foods according to directions, leaving out the salt when you are processing them. They will keep just as well as vegetables canned using salt.

It is important that you use the latest information when you are canning vegetables, since research has shown that it is better to process foods for a longer time than we used to think was necessary. Vegetables, except for tomatoes, should be canned in a pressure canner. Information on that process is available from the manufacturers of the canners, your county extension agent, the makers of canning jars, and numerous other publications.

The only food that needs salt when it is being prepared is pickles. That is not because the salt helps preserve the pickles, but because the salt draws water out of the vegetables, which is then replaced with sugar and vinegar to make them crisp and flavorful. There are recipes for making pickles without salt, but they must be kept in the refrigerator and are not good canned.

You can prepare pickles without sugar, if you like. In fact, one large company is now selling diabetic pickles in the stores and they are very good. Dill pickles are made without sugar and are readily available, but I prefer a sweet pickle. I worked on making a sweet pickle that I liked, and finally came up with a couple that I think you might like also—so I have included them at the end of this chapter.

Freezing fruits and vegetables is sometimes simpler than canning them. We generally think of fruits as being frozen with sugar, but they also freeze very well without it. During the summer I always prepare applesauce, cooked rhubarb, and other cooked fruits and freeze them. Then I add sugar substitute when I am ready to use them. You can also freeze uncooked fruits for use during the winter when they aren't available (or at least they aren't available in small towns like Wadena).

Fruits may be frozen in their own juices or in water to which an antidarkening agent such as citric or ascorbic acid has been added. Gooseberries, currants, cranberries, blueberries, and rhubarb freeze well in freezer bags or containers just as they are without any liquid or antidarkening agents. Some other fruits may be frozen individually on wax paper-lined cookie sheets and then bagged in a freezer bag after they are frozen. Fruits that we especially like this way include strawberries, raspberries, blueberries, and huckleberries. Of course, all of these fruits are washed well before they are frozen. The only fruit that shouldn't be washed before freezing is cranberries, and the directions on the wrapper for cranberries tell you this. We wash fruits well, drain them well (by lifting them out of the water instead of pouring the water off of them), lay them on wax paper, and pop them into the coldest part of the freezer for several hours until they are completely frozen. The reason they should be frozen in the coldest part of the freezer, and as rapidly as possible, is that if you freeze them slowly larger ice crystals will develop and the texture won't be as good when they are defrosted.

If you don't grow your own fresh fruit (and not too many people do), it is fun to buy it at wayside stands, open air markets, and sometimes from your friends and neighbors. Some stores will order fruit for you frozen in larger quantities without sugar. We buy it this way and then bag it in smaller bags to put in the freezer. This way we can get fresh fruits that aren't available to us here, such as Bing cherries and Royal Ann cherries.

Fruit that is packed in freezer bags should have as much of the air squeezed out as possible. Leave ½ inch for expansion in rigid freezer containers. The fruit should be labelled with the name of the fruit and the date and any other information you want to add. Frozen fruit should be stored at zero degrees or lower and used within 8–12 months for best quality. Unsweetened fruits lose quality faster than those sweetened with sugar or syrup. Partially defrosted fruits taste best to me, although they have to be fully defrosted if they are to be used in salad. Fruit may be defrosted at room temperature in the freezing container. If faster defrosting is necessary, submerge the container in lukewarm water until defrosted or defrost in a microwave.

MRS. RILEY'S PICKLES

Yields 7 quarts or 14 pints

This recipe is based on that old standby, 14-day pickles. We call them Mrs. Riley's pickles because my cousin Virginia Ballantine's grandmother, Mrs. Riley, used to make them every year. Virginia's family doesn't care for them so she doesn't make them; however, they are Chuck's and my favorite pickles and I have continued to make them—the sweet version for Chuck and this diabetic version for me—and I honestly like mine just as well as his.

Make only enough for one year because they are wonderful the first year—sweet, spicy, and crisp—but they lose some of their quality the second year.

2½ quarts vinegar
2 cups sugar
2 tablespoons celery seed
1 ounce stick cinnamon
10 drops green or red vegetable coloring (optional)
2 gallons washed and sliced medium-size firm cucumbers with the ends removed
1 gallon boiling water
2 cups pickling salt
1 gallon boiling water (day 7)
1 gallon boiling water (day 9)
1 tablespoon alum
1 gallon boiling water (day 10)
Sugar substitute equal to 1½ cups sugar

Heat together vinegar, sugar, celery seed, cinnamon, and vegetable coloring. Cool to room temperature and return to the vinegar container. Cover tightly and let set until needed. (I like to use some coloring because it enhances the color of the pickles and makes them look more like the commercial sweet pickle slices. I sometimes make a red batch for gifts and to use on relish trays on special occasions.)

Place cucumbers in empty glass gallon jars, stainless steel pots, or crocks. Dissolve pickling salt in 1 gallon boiling water and then pour over cucumbers. Let stand, covered loosely, for 1 week. Remove any mold on top of the cucumbers at the end of 7 days.

On the seventh day, drain pickles well. Pour 1 gallon boiling water over them and let them set, covered loosely, for 2 days.

On the ninth day, drain cucumbers well. Dissolve the alum in 1 gallon boiling water and pour over cucumbers.

On the tenth day, drain pickles well and cover with 1 gallon boiling water. On the eleventh day, drain cucumbers well and pack into 7 quart or 14 pint sterilized jars.

Strain the reserved vinegar mixture. Throw away the spices and heat the vinegar. Add sugar substitute and pour over the sliced cucumbers in the jars. (Do not use NutraSweet or Equal [aspartame] since it is not stable to heat.) Cover and seal the jars. Process in a hot water bath 10 minutes for pints and 15 minutes for quarts. Serve 2 tablespoons per serving.

Nutritive values per serving:	CAL	CHO (gm)	PRO (gm)	FAT (gm)	NA (mg)
	9	1	negl.	negl.	264

Food exchanges per serving: Up to ¼ cup may be considered free
Low-sodium diets: This recipe is not suitable.

ZUCCHINI PICKLES

Yields 5 pints—80 servings

There are so many zucchini around that I thought I'd try to make some pickles from them. I used the recipe that I always use for bread and butter pickles and it really worked well. Everyone liked them very much.

1 gallon thinly sliced 6- to 8-inch-long zucchini
4 cups sliced white onions
½ cup salt
2 quarts cracked ice
5 cups cider vinegar
3 cups water
1½ teaspoons tumeric
1 teaspoon celery seed
1 tablespoon mustard seed
Sugar substitute to taste

Combine zucchini, onions, salt, and ice in a large bowl and mix well. Cover with a plate with a weight on top of it so that all of the zucchini slices are covered with the salted ice water formed as the ice melts. Let them set for 3 hours and then drain them well. Place in a large saucepan.

Thoroughly mix vinegar, water, tumeric, celery seed, and mustard seed and add to zucchini. Bring almost to a boil but do not let mixture boil, stirring frequently with a wooden spoon. Pack the hot pickles in pint jars.

Add sugar substitute to taste to the hot liquid. I use about ¼ cup of liquid sugar substitute, but you may prefer them a little sweeter or even a little less sweet. Pour the hot liquid over the pickles to about ½ inch from the top. Cover and seal. Process in a hot water bath for 5 minutes. (Do not use Equal [aspartame] to sweeten the pickles because it is not stable to heat and the pickles are processed in a hot water bath.) Serve 2 tablespoons pickles per serving.

Nutritive values per serving:	CAL	CHO (gm)	PRO (gm)	FAT (gm)	NA (mg)
	8	1	negl.	negl.	*

Food exchanges per serving: Up to ¼ cup may be considered free
Low-sodium diets: This recipe is not suitable.

*varies

FROZEN SLICED SWEET DILL PICKLES

Yields 1 quart—16 servings

This recipe is from Nellie Yurkovich, who like us retired here in Wadena. She had lived all over the world with her career army husband, Tony, who died in 1976. After his death she returned to Wadena, where she had lived as a child and young woman.

1 pound 3-inch unwaxed cucumbers
2 cups packed, sliced yellow onions
4 teaspoons salt
2 tablespoons water
¼ cup sugar
1 tablespoon Weight Watchers dry sugar substitute
½ cup white vinegar
¼ cup garlic wine vinegar
1 tablespoon dry dill weed

Wash cucumbers and slice them about ⅛ inch thick. Place cucumbers, onions, salt, and water in a 2-quart glass or stainless-steel bowl (don't use aluminum) and let stand for 2 hours at room temperature or overnight in the refrigerator. Drain cucumbers and onions, but do not rinse.

Combine sugar, sugar substitute, vinegars, and dill weed. Stir until sugar is dissolved and then add vegetables. The liquid should cover vegetables. Cover and refrigerate 2 hours.

Pack pickles lightly in jars or plastic containers, leaving 1 inch at top for expansion. Seal tightly and freeze. The pickles may be kept in the freezer for 6 months. Use within 3 or 4 days after defrosting. Two days of freezing is enough if you want to use them right away. Use ¼ cup per serving.

Nutritive values per serving:	CAL	CHO (gm)	PRO (gm)	FAT (gm)	NA (mg)
	24	6	negl.	negl.	534

Food exchanges per serving: 1 vegetable
Low-sodium diets: Rinse pickles after they are drained before vinegar is added.

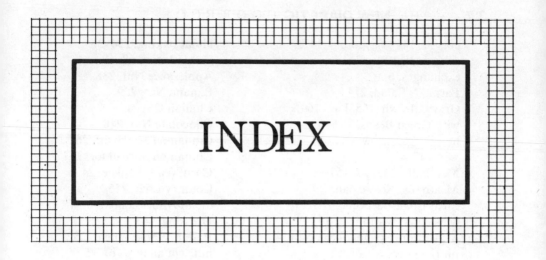

INDEX